www.harcourt-international.com

Bringing you products from all Harcourt Health Sciences companies including Baillière Tindall, Churchill Livingstone, Mosby and W.B. Saunders

- ▶ **Browse** for latest information on new books, journals and electronic products

- ▶ **Search** for information on over 20 000 published titles with full product information including tables of contents and sample chapters

- ▶ **Keep up to date** with our extensive publishing programme in your field by registering with eAlert or requesting postal updates

- ▶ **Secure online ordering** with prompt delivery, as well as full contact details to order by phone, fax or post

- ▶ **News** of special features and promotions

If you are based in the following countries, please visit the country-specific site to receive full details of product availability and local ordering information

USA: www.harcourthealth.com

Canada: www.harcourtcanada.com

Australia: www.harcourt.com.au

🌸 Baillière Tindall   Mosby   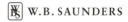 W.B. SAUNDERS

Understanding the Placebo Effect in Complementary Medicine

For Churchill Livingstone:

Publishing Manager: Inta Ozols
Project Development Manager: Katrina Mather
Project Manager: Derek Robertson
Design Direction: George Ajayi

Understanding the Placebo Effect in Complementary Medicine
Theory, Practice and Research

Edited by

David Peters MB ChB DRCOG MFHom MRO
**Clinical Director, The Centre for Community Care and Primary Health,
University of Westminster, London, UK**

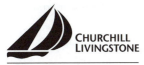

EDINBURGH LONDON NEW YORK PHILADELPHIA ST LOUIS SYDNEY TORONTO 2001

CHURCHILL LIVINGSTONE
An imprint of Harcourt Publishers Limited

© Harcourt Publishers Limited 2001

 is a registered trademark of Harcourt Publishers Limited

The right of David Peters to be identified as editor of this work has
been asserted by him in accordance with the Copyright, Designs and
Patents Act 1988.

First published 2001
 Reprinted 2001

ISBN 0443 06031 2

British Library Cataloguing in Publication Data
A catalogue record for this book is available from the British Library

Library of Congress Cataloging in Publication Data
A catalog record for this book is available from the Library of
Congress

Note
Medical knowledge is constantly changing. As new information
becomes available, changes in treatment, procedures, equipment and
the use of drugs become necessary. The editor, contributors and the
publishers have taken care to ensure that the information given in this
text is accurate and up to date. However, readers are strongly advised
to confirm that the information, especially with regard to drug usage,
complies with the latest legislation and standards of practice.

The
publisher's
policy is to use
**paper manufactured
from sustainable forests**

Printed in China by RDC Group Limited
C/02

Contents

Contributors

Angela Clow PhD
Senior Lecturer, Department of Psychology,
University of Westminster, London, UK

Anton J M de Craen PhD
Clinical Epidemiologist, Department of Clinical Epidemiology,
Leiden University Medical Centre, The Netherlands

Edzard Ernst MD PhD
Director, Department of Complementary Medicine,
University of Exeter, Exeter, UK

Peter Fenwick MB BChir(Cantab) DPM FRCPsych
Consultant Neuropsychiatrist Emeritus, Maudsley Hospital, London, UK

James Hawkins MB BChir(Cantab)
Independent Specialist, Edinburgh, UK

Cecil G Helman MB ChB MRCGP DipSocAnthrop
Associate Professor, Department of Human Sciences,
Brunel University, Uxbridge, UK;
Senior Lecturer, Department of Primary Care and Population Sciences,
Royal Free and University College Medical School, London, UK

John Heron BA
Director, South Pacific Centre for Human Inquiry,
Auckland, New Zealand

Dr med **Helmut Keine**
Institut für angewandte Erkenntnistheorie and medizinische
Methodologie, Bad Krozingen, Germany

Dr med **Gunver S Kienle**
Institut für angewandte Erkenntnistheorie and medizinische
Methodologie, Bad Krozingen, Germany

Jos Kleijen MD PhD
Professor and Director, NHS Centre for Reviews and Dissemination,
University of York, York, UK

Phil Latey DO
Private Practitioner and Lecturer, Sydney, Australia

Angela J E M Lampe-Schoenmaeckers MD
Anesthesiologist, Department of Anesthesiology, Academic Medical
Centre, University of Amsterdam, Amsterdam, The Netherlands

David Reilly FRCP MRCGP FFHom
Consultant Physician, Glasgow Homoeopathic Hospital, Glasgow, UK;
Honorary Senior Lecturer in Medicine, University of Glasgow,
Glasgow, UK

Janet Richardson PhD BSc RN DipDN PGCE RNT
Director of Integrated Health Development, School of Health Care,
Oxford Brookes University, Oxford, UK

Jean Sayre-Adams RN MA RPTT
Director, The Sacred Space Foundation, Cumbria, UK

Robert Withers MPhil BAc RSHom
Private Practitioner; Senior Lecturer, University of Westminster,
London, UK

Stephen G Wright MSc RN RNT DipN DANS RPTT FRCN MBE
Associate Professor, Faculty of Health, St Martin's College, Lancaster, UK;
Chairman, The Scared Space Foundation, Cumbria, UK;

Preface

Complementary practitioners promote the idea that their methods somehow 'switch on' self-organising processes. One of complementary and alternative medicine's most intriguing implications for mainstream health care is that doctors should re-integrate this aspect of the healing task; that we must not only confront established pathology but also learn how better to catalyse the process of healing. As practitioners we prefer to think we are effective: why else would we be practitioners? But therein lie several potential problems: firstly, because we might be less effective than we like to think; and secondly, that therefore it will be difficult to reflect honestly on our effectiveness. In the search to become more effective some practitioners aim for ever more technical expertise, but to what extent is our therapeutic effectiveness determined by our humanity and presence rather than technical knowledge and our skill as a therapist? How much of a treatment's effect is due the patients own response and resilience? Would it be demeaning if we as practitioners had to accept that a great deal of recovery depends on responses we trigger and, that as practitioners we have to persuade, rather than force recovery?

In everyday speech, a placebo is a fake treatment, something given to please the patient. How strange then that placebo effects should be so strong; so consistent that experimental studies must be intricately designed to avoid them, so great is their influence on treatment outcomes. Modern clinical trials aim to bracket off all human variables and bias by using randomisation and blinding, for only when they achieve this, can small differences in outcome between experimental group and control group be attributed to the treatment alone. Yet the fact that around 60% of control groups tend to improve forces us to ask what the personal and inter-personal factors that so profoundly affect outcomes might be; and how we should make better use of them. There are important issues here: why are 'fake' treatments so effective and so hard to distinguish from 'real' ones; what ought we to make of the insidious implication that personal and inter-personal elements are not part of proper practice? Since they include resilience, natural remission and the effect of a good practitioner-client relationship – all desirable aspects of good medicine – these 'human factors' ought surely to be understood and maximised rather than excluded. In reality, of course, these elements are an inseparable part of practice, for we do not work in a vacuum and the art of communication has its proper place in all professional life. Over-reliance on technique and an inability to engage humanly is arguably a sign of practitioner boredom, burn-out and depression.

The placebo response focuses our mind on health care as a skilled human activity, so it is of particular interest to those of us whose clinical work involves skilled use of hands, heart or language. In fact, complementary therapies and psychotherapies have proven very hard to fit into the framework of randomised controlled trials; so has family medicine. I believe the insinuation that they are therefore unscientific and that hard science alone should be a basis for proper practice has harmed health care by diminishing the 'art of medicine'. The over-emphasis on technical effectiveness has also sidelined medicine's interest in our innate capacity for natural recovery and made us all less curious about how to support them. Lately, however, because medical technology has met with only limited success in treating epidemic chronic degenerative diseases, the question of how to catalyse resilience has come to the fore.

In the 1970s, when George Engel made his famous challenge to biomedicine and set out a framework for a bio-psycho-social model, these bio-psychological pathways were still ill-defined. Nowadays psychophysiology has better maps and it is widely acknowledged that psycho-social pressures are met by physiological and potentially pathophysiological changes; we can cite clear examples of beneficial psychosomatic effects. Obviously then human factors do have a powerful influence on health, health care and all treatments. So, to dismiss this as mere placebo response and at best the result of pious fraud is no longer satisfactory. Any practitioner who thinks about her work will rightly feel some uncertainty about how her presence and personality *as well as* the treatments she gives, affects her patients. But by mixing up and confusing these and other influences, the concept of placebo effect may well have undermined our confidence in humane practice and quite possibly made it more difficult.

With these questions in mind a conference was held at the University of Westminster in collaboration with the Scientific and Medical Network in September 1997. This book builds on some leading thoughts presented there. The conference brought practitioners and researchers together around the theme of self-healing responses and the keynote address was given by Professor Herbert Benson, whose *Timeless healing: the power and biology of belief* (Benson & Stark 1996), had been published just before the conference. Our own book is one ripple in the wave of renewed interest Benson's book heralded. Important contributions to our understanding made since include books by Harrington (1997) and by Dixon and Sweeney

(2000) The Harrington book arose out of a fascinating Harvard Conference in 1994 and it updates in important ways the key work on placebo response, the ground-breaking book *Placebo–theory research and mechanisms* (White et al 1985). Dixon and Sweeney's book (2000) has set out to rehabilitate and re-value human and contextual factors, warning against the dangers of losing them from clinical practice. We hope our collection of accounts from practice will complement these works.

This book is for practitioners who want to think about the balance between technique and relationship in their own work. Our authors offer theoretical frameworks from psychology, psycho-immunology and anthropology, but there can be no single explanation or final word written on this topic. For, given the great array of influences on treatment outcomes, a single general theory of health and healing would be impossible to achieve. Nor would it be desirable. Alongside various theoretical perspectives you will find here chapters by practitioners with diverse clinical perspectives who have thought about how non-technical factors (being with, rather than doing to patients) influence their own practice. These are highly experienced voices: at times highly subjective, idiosyncratic and convinced. Any authority they carry depends on their authenticity, and these accounts are presented here as reflective work-in-progress. They are an attempt to share the maps and imaginations practitioners use to make sense of their experience of what happens in the space between themselves and their clients. As such they are about belief and being, rather than fact. We expect them to be wondered about, questioned and criticised by colleagues, with the aim of reaching beyond out current understanding of the inter-subjective world and how it might influence healing outcomes.

The human self-healing response is a realm where the boundaries between subjective mind and objective body blur and fade. How could we learn to use it wisely and well? Our authors offer some ideas about this. How might we, as practitioners and scientists, reflect on this elusive capacity for self-healing and our role in it as therapists? Two very different approaches to research are discussed: one experimental and searching for objectivity, the other qualitative and searching for a rigorous subjectivity. No doubt both these approaches and more too, will be needed as we unfold a new science of health.

Lydia Temoshok (1986) has compared the term 'placebo' to a theory used by 18th century chemists, who, before oxidation was understood, postulated a burning substance loses 'phlogiston'. Because the notion appeared to fit some of the facts, it delayed the discovery of oxygen and the acceptance of the true explanation – oxidation. Similarly, the placebo concept hides our ignorance and perpetuates partial truths about clinical work and outcomes while at the same time obscuring a better understanding. Is the placebo response our phlogiston? Will it disappear from our language once we have a real grasp of the therapeutic relationship and mind-body interactions? We hope this book casts some light on these questions and inspires practitioners to reflect on their own and their clients' humanity and the extra-ordinary human capacity for self-healing.

London, 2001   David Peters

REFERENCES

Benson H, Stark M 1996 Timeless healing: the power and biology of belief. Scribner, New York

Dixon M, Sweeney K 2000 The human effect in medicine: theory, research and practice. Radcliffe Medical Press, Oxford

Harrington A (ed) 1997 The placebo effect: an interdisciplinary exploration. Harvard University Press, Cambridge, MA

Temoshok L 1986 Review of Placebo – theory, research and mechanisms. Advances in Mind-Body Medicine 3(1): 71–73

White L, Tursky B, Schwartz G (eds) 1985 Placebo – theory, research and mechanisms. Guilford Press, New York

SECTION 1

Theory

SECTION CONTENTS

Placebos and nocebos: the cultural construction of belief

Cecil G. Helman

Editor's note

Cecil Helman's book 'Culture, health and illness' made me aware that our 'obvious' ways of doing medicine actually depend on a hidden world view, a framework of unexamined assumptions that holds our thinking in place. When looked at through the anthropologist's eye, many deeply rooted certainties (including mind–body dualism and a bias towards reductionism) can be seen for what they are: beliefs. I wanted Hellman's anthropological gaze to liberate us from the notion of real and unreal elements in treatment. One wrong assumption we make is that placebos are 'things' that fool us into feeling better. In this chapter he persuades us that the greater part of any treatment outcome has to do with factors that are anything but biological. Even apparently unequivocal clinical facts actually depend on culture and custom; in fact, even within the practice of conventional medicine in Europe, diagnoses, treatments and symptom patterns vary from nation to nation. He helps us see that the way we think about health and healthcare is culture bound—making it obvious for instance that, at a time when beliefs and social relationships are changing, people will seek out new ways of putting together their healing encounters, and making it seem less strange that effectiveness and beliefs should be so intricately bound together. Hellman not only gives us a framework for asking how and why complementary therapies have taken such a hold, but also calls into question whether treatment, relationships and outcomes can ever be fully understood if plucked out of their cultural landscape.

There are many different ways of understanding the placebo effect: this chapter deals with some of the perspectives of *social anthropology*. Anthropology is the study, and comparison, of different human groups, societies and cultures—particularly of their social organization, beliefs and behaviours. An editorial in the British Medical Journal (Editorial 1980) has called it 'the most scientific of the humanities and the most humane of the sciences'. One recent branch of social anthropology, *medical anthropology*, is the study of how people in different cultural and social groups explain the causes of ill health, the types of treatment they believe in and the people and institutions to whom they turn if they do get ill. It is also concerned with how these health-related beliefs and behaviours relate to physical, psychological and social changes in the human organism, in both health and disease (Helman 2000).

THE ROLE OF CONTEXT IN PLACEBO AND NOCEBO PHENOMENONA

The concepts of medical anthropology are particularly relevant to under-standing the role of *context* in the placebo and nocebo phenomena—that is, the extent to which both are influenced by the social, cultural, economic and physical environment in which they appear. Of key importance are the mechanisms by which certain human groups—whether societies or cultural groups—create, reinforce and maintain the belief system that underlies these phenomena.

To the anthropologist, placebos and nocebos are always, to some extent, *culture bound*, for they do not exist in a vacuum. Their effects always depend, to some degree, on the wider context of cultural beliefs, values, expectations, assumptions and norms as well as on certain social and economic realities in which they occur. All of these help to create belief in the placebo in the first place: validating both its healing power and that of the person who actually administers it. This implies, therefore, that placebos that work in one cultural group may not necessarily have the same effect in another.

THE 'TOTAL DRUG EFFECT'

One model developed by Claridge (1970) in psychopharmacology provides a useful way of conceptualizing some aspects of the placebo effect. He suggested the concept of the 'total drug effect' whereby the overall effect of a drug on an individual usually depends on a number of different factors in addition to (or separate from) its pharmacological action. These are the attributes of: (1) the *drug* itself (such as its colour, shape, form, brand name and price), (2) the *prescriber* (such as attitude, beliefs, self-confidence, air of authority and clothing), (3) the *recipient* (such as psychological state,

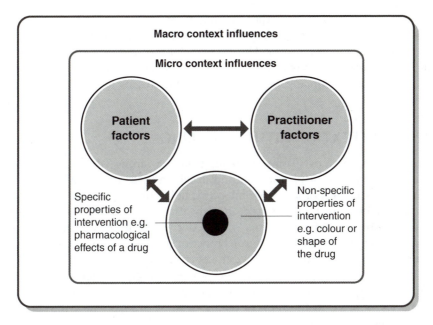

Figure 1.1 A medical anthropological model of factors influencing the placebo response.

suggestibility, intelligence and personality), and (4) the *setting* or physical environment in which prescribing or ingestion takes place (physical environments such as home, clinic or hospital). In this model, therefore, the purest form of the placebo effect would be the total drug effect—but *without* the pharmacological presence of any drug.

In Figure 1.1 is my adapted version of this model expressed in diagrammatic form, but with a greater emphasis on the role of context. This has two interrelated aspects: (1) the *microcontext* (Claridge's 'setting'), and (2) the *macrocontext* in which it is embedded. The latter refers to the wider social, cultural and economic milieu in which prescribing, and ingestion, take place. Both forms of context are crucial means by which different societies and cultures create an ambience, or atmosphere, in which belief in the efficacy of a healer and of their treatments (whether placebo or not) can be created, maximized and then maintained over time. They not only influence the prescriber and recipient, and their attitudes towards the drug, but also help create belief in the minds of the recipient's family and friends, and of other spectators.

In medical anthropology, the concept of 'placebo effect' is not confined only to medications: to chemically inactive substances used in double-blind studies. It includes any 'pill, potion or procedure' (Wolf 1959) where belief plays an important part. This is because all forms of healing—

whether medical or non-medical, orthodox or complementary, modern or traditional—make use of this phenomenon to some extent. Even when a treatment does have a physical basis (as in surgery, radiotherapy or the use of medications), there is always likely to be some element of the placebo effect as well: enhancing belief, and expectations, in the efficacy of that treatment.

THE CONTEXT OF RITUAL HEALING

Cross-culturally, most forms of healing have a strong ritual component. The 'microcontext' or physical setting in which these rituals takes place—whether a doctor's office, hospital ward, holy shrine or house of a traditional healer—can be compared to a theatre set complete with scenery, props, costumes and script. This 'script', derived from the culture ('macrocontext') itself, is usually known to most of the participants. It tells them how to behave, how to experience the event and what to expect from it. It helps to validate the healer, and the power of their methods of healing. Thus the physical setting itself is never neutral. It always contributes, in some subtle way, to the totality of the healing process—and thus to the placebo effect as well.

A vital component of this process is the use of *ritual symbols*. Most forms of healing, in different communities, employ a whole cluster of these symbols. They may be not only specific objects, equipment, documents or decorations but also certain standardized types of body language, movement, posture, dance, clothing, speech and sound. In some cases, they may also include music, songs or communal chants, and even the use of different scents (such as temple or church incense).

In each case, they have a specific purpose: not so much practical as symbolic. Their main role is to create an appropriate ambience for the placebo effect. They are there to transmit important information to clients, and to those around them, about the healer, the techniques, frame of reference, and cultural sources of the healing power (whether it is medical science, Ayurveda, Traditional Chinese Medicine, or any other). From an anthropological perspective, most of the symbols used in rituals of healing have this function. As Turner (1969) remarks of the symbols used in the healing rituals of the Ndembu people of Zambia, 'almost every article used, every gesture employed, every song or prayer, every unit of space and time, by convention stands for something other than itself'. Each symbol used in such a ritual acts as a 'storage unit' into which is packed the maximum amount of information about the basic cultural premises of that society (Turner 1968). At times of illness, danger, transition and uncertainty, transmission of such information is crucial—for it comprises ways of restating, and communicating, the basic premises of everyday life: of reassuring sick, unhappy or confused people that despite their suffering the world still 'makes sense' and is as it always was. And that, too, is an essential component of the placebo effect.

Not all of the available symbols may actually be used in any particular healing ritual. Some of them, such as the elaborate diplomas on a physician's wall, or the rows of impressive-looking books on the shelf, will have no practical function in either consultation or treatment. They act more like catalysts: essential to a particular process, but without being actively involved in it. Like other components of the 'total drug effect', their function is to 'set the scene' and help create belief and expectations in the minds of all concerned.

Thus, for the medical anthropologist, a deeper understanding of any placebo effect—whether medical or not—must involve the 'decoding' of the messages hidden within the rituals and symbols associated with it. To understand the placebo effect fully is to understand the society in which it occurs. This is because the symbols that help sustain it are both derived from, and validated by, the wider sociocultural milieu (or 'macrocontext')—and help to validate it in turn.

CONTEXTS OF RITUAL HEALING: SOME EXAMPLES

Both medical anthropology and medical history provide many examples of how practitioners, in different places and at different times, have sought to create this effect, and the types of ritual symbols that they have employed.

Traditional healers

In much of the non-Western world, the leading practitioners of the placebo effect are traditional healers. These include the various types of shaman and diviner found in many countries, such as the *curanderos* of Latin America, the *sangomas* of Southern Africa, the *tang-kis* of Taiwan, the healers of the Brazilian *Umbanda* cult and numerous others. Like Western doctors, all these work within a specific context—both physical and socio-cultural—employing certain techniques, rituals and symbols, and a certain use of time and place, in order to enhance belief in their healing powers and practices.

Even when these healers do utilize physical treatments (such as herbs, potions or massage) they seem to be more aware of the positive powers of belief than Western doctors. Often they regard their patient's belief system as an essential ally in the treatment, rather than as an enemy: as something intrinsic to any act of healing, which needs to be exploited. As a result they are more willing to involve actively patients, their family and their community in the various rituals of treatment (Martin 1981). By contrast, many Western doctors prefer to view their patients as more passive—and medical textbooks and journals commonly sneer at what they describe as 'just a placebo effect': a peripheral phenomenon which they cannot easily measure, predict or explain, and which therefore is not quite 'real'.

Setting

The setting in which a traditional healer works may be a shrine, a temple, a church, the tomb of a holy saint, a sacred place of pilgrimage or a special room in their own house. Within these different contexts, the ritual symbols used are often syncretic in origin combining ritual symbols from several different healing traditions for maximum effect. They may include certain sacred objects, fetishes, holy texts, books, idols, icons, relics and special paintings, as well as medical items. Mull (1983), for example, describes the consulting room of a Mexican–American *curandero*, or folk healer, in southern California, which blends both medical and religious imagery. In addition to bookshelves filled with medical reference books, and a 2-foot high synthetic skeleton, the walls are hung with numerous large religious paintings of Christ on the Cross, and the Last Supper, as well as an ornate sombrero and a guitar.

Traditional healers often make skilful use of their consultation times to enhance belief, and improve cooperation. Kleinman (1978, 1980) describes how consultations with the *tang-ki*, the shaman and traditional healer of Taiwan, usually take place in a small temple or shrine decorated with both Taoist and Buddhist images. Adorned with sacred artefacts and smelling of incense, its centre is dominated by a large, impressive altar upon which are placed small painted wooden figures of various other deities associated with the shrine. The shaman is surrounded by a group of helpers, often makes diagnoses while in a trance and always wears a special cloak with a bright red sash. Consultations with a *tang-ki* last only 5–10 minutes, but the entire time is spent in explaining the disease and its treatment to the patient. By contrast, Western-style doctors on Taiwan spend only 40 seconds giving such explanations to their patients (Kleinman 1978).

El-Islam (1982) too describes how in some Arab countries ill people often visit religious figures and shrines to be healed, as well as consulting a doctor. These may include the tombs of a famous sheikh or master (*Al-Asyaad*). In many cases, there is also the use of amulets or holy verses by patients, and rituals of purification (*Mahuw* or *Mahaya*). Some traditional healers supply amulets containing holy texts, or advise the patient to drink or wash in water that has previously been washed off koranic verses.

Explanation of the illness

Explaining why the person got ill is an essential part of most traditional and religious healing. While Western doctors spend their time telling patients what has happened ('your artery has blocked up', 'your kidney isn't working'), these healers try to supply answers to the questions seriously ill people often ask: 'Why has it happened?', 'Why to me?', 'Why now?', 'What have I done to deserve it?' or even: 'Who has *caused* me to be ill?' They may relate the illness to people's prior moral behaviour, their spiritual status, or their failure to pray or to appease their ancestors. In these cases, 'prayer and repentance, not penicillin, cure sin' (Snow 1978). In each case, this type of concentrated, individualized attention—as well as the use of certain ritual symbols—helps to create the right atmosphere for the placebo effect.

Western medicine

Even though based on science, modern medicine also makes considerable efforts to create, or enhance, the placebo effect. The consulting rooms, surgeries and wards of Western medicine are adorned with many ritual symbols that do not take part in the consultation itself but help create an atmosphere of belief, expectation and trust in the doctor's healing powers. These symbols may include: elaborate diplomas on the wall (often written in Latin); rows of large books on a shelf; cases of elaborate, shiny instruments and equipment; adverts for pharmaceutical products; uniformed and deferential helpers, such as nurses or receptionists; the faint smells of disinfectant; and so on. Combined with formal dress, grooming, manner, body language and way of speaking, all of these help create the appropriate ambience. They also transmit to the patient a message about the healing powers of medical science, and of this particular representative of it. In that sense, they are an important part of the 'total drug effect'.

In Western medicine, the doctor's white coat is one of the most potent of all ritual symbols. Although its function is ostensibly to maintain cleanliness and hygiene, it also acts as a powerful symbol: a crucial component of the placebo effect. It can be regarded as what Turner (1968) terms a 'multivocal symbol': that is, one that transmits many different messages at the same time. What does it tell us about the person who wears it? Elsewhere (Helman 2000) I have listed some of its cluster of meanings. They include: a special training and licence to practise medicine; familiarity with the situations of illness, suffering and death; reliability and efficiency; a scientific orientation; a commitment to caring, and the relief of suffering; respectability and high social status; and sexual neutrality. It also stands for the *power* to ask intimate questions, examine patients' bodies, make life and death decisions, prescribe tests and medications and—if necessary—confine people against their will to mental and other hospitals. Like all ritual symbols, the doctor's white coat draws much of its symbolic power from the context in which it is worn. For this reason, it has a very different effect on patients from that worn by the laboratory technician, the pharmacist, the medical receptionist, the beautician or the supermarket salesperson.

Like all ritual symbols used to mobilize the placebo effect, it may sometimes have just the opposite effect: as in 'white coat hypertension' (Long et al 1990), or 'white coat hyperglycaemia' (Campbell et al 1992).

Cultural differences

Modern medicine is not culturally homogeneous, and the consulting rooms of physicians from different backgrounds often utilize very different symbols to create the right atmosphere.

In the USA, for example, both specialists and family physicians often wear white coats in their offices. Unlike in Britain, it is also quite common for the walls to be adorned with impressive diplomas, certificates, degrees, plaques, prizes and commendations. Like the images, icons and other props of the traditional healer these help create belief and expectations in the minds of patients: a public, symbolic display of the healing powers, professional success and legitimacy of this particular practitioner of modern medicine.

In Britain, by contrast, the creation of this placebo atmosphere seems to draw more on the symbolic powers of class, hierarchy and affluence. The rooms of a Harley Street specialist, for example, tend to have a more restrained display of diplomas. Power derives, to some extent, from the prestigious address itself; from certain types of very formal clothing, body language and accent; from the deference of receptionists, nurses and other patients; from the size, furnishings and decorations of the waiting room— with its thick carpets, hunting prints and copies of *Country Life*, *Tatler* and *House and Garden* lying on tables; and from the knowledge that the consultation itself will be lengthy, exclusive and very expensive.

The psychoanalyst

Psychoanalysis, like all forms of 'talk therapy', takes great pains to create the correct atmosphere for its healing sessions. The office of Sigmund Freud, founder of psychoanalysis, has been re-created at the Freud Museum in London, with the original furnishings, paintings and ornaments brought from Vienna. It too is adorned with symbols that transmit a clear and powerful message of Freud's background, areas of interests, professional success and ideology of healing to the patient. It is dominated not by the altar or shrine of a *tang-ki*, but by his large desk and the sacred couch, covered with rich textiles, on which his clients would lie and talk. The room's shelves are lined with many artefacts from ancient Rome, Greece and Egypt. Collectively, these can be regarded as ritual symbols. Not only do they help create a particular atmosphere, but they also transmit messages about Freud's interest in psychic archaeology. For, as he once remarked, the psychoanalyst's work 'resembles to a great extent an archaeologist's excavation of some dwelling-place that has been destroyed or buried' (McDougall 1989). They may help create a scene that was indispensable for his particular type of psychological healing.

Anton Mesmer

In medical history, one of the most famous practitioners of the placebo art was probably the faith healer, Friedrich Anton Mesmer (1734–1815). He believed that the universe was dominated by 'magnetic forces' whose disturbance was the sole cause of all disease. Many of the symbols and techniques that he used were drawn from science, but interpreted in his own special way. He claimed to have cured many people with convulsions, paralyses, hysteria, headaches, blindness and 'congestion' of the liver and spleen. Rose (1971) describes the scene at one of his healing seances:

In a large room well supplied with mirrors, flowers, stained glass and incense, sufferers were put into a receptive frame of mind by soft music. In the centre was a tub filled with iron filings, from which protruded rods; round this the patients sat in silent circles, holding either the ends of the rods or each others' hands. At the critical moment the 'magnetist' himself came in, dressed in a silk robe and holding yet another iron rod. He then passed around the circle, staring into his patients' eyes, touching them or making passes over them.

As he did so, many of the patients would swoon, or go into a trance, from which they would later awake—fully 'cured'.

THE MACROCONTEXT OF WESTERN MEDICINE

To understand the placebos used in modern society, especially those prescribed by doctors, one needs to understand the cultural 'macrocontext' that validates them. Like traditional healing, modern medicine itself does not exist in a cultural vacuum. It too is the concentrated expression of a much wider belief system: of the values, beliefs and expectations of the society in which it occurs. Increasingly, this is the belief in the power and efficacy of *medications*, prescribed by doctor, nurse or pharmacist—or self-prescribed. This belief in healing chemicals is an essential component of Western forms of the placebo effect.

Over the past century or so, there seems to have been a major cultural shift in Western society. It is in the types, and amounts, of 'chemical comforters' (Claridge 1970) that are used to improve daily life, reduce individual suffering and solve many personal problems. In addition to the continuing use of alcohol, tobacco and opiates, there has been a shift towards medically prescribed psychotropic drugs: tranquillizers, antidepressants and sleeping tablets. According to Joyce (1969) part of their effect depends, also, on the placebo phenomenon. The cultural 'macrocontext' of contemporary society is therefore one of progressive *normalization* of what has been called 'pills for personal problems' (Trethowan 1975). To Warburton (1978) we are in danger of becoming a 'pharmacotopia' where 'chemical coping' (Pellegrino 1976) becomes a predominant way of dealing with the vicissitudes of daily life. This growing emphasis on the 'chemical road to success'—whether legal or illegal chemicals—has become a major cultural background to the placebo effect. There are now a wide variety of 'chemical comforters' available. They range from more socially acceptable ones—such as tea, coffee, alcohol, tobacco, snuff, chocolate, tonics, bitters, vitamins, herbal preparations, over-the-counter patent remedies and medically prescribed psychotropic drugs—to illegal drugs such as marijuana, heroin, ecstasy, LSD and crack cocaine.

Perhaps as a result of our increasingly isolated, individualistic lives the overall cultural model seems to be that of 'incomplete individuals': people who need to 'complete' themselves, with the aid of a chemical, in order to function in a more successful way. Without it, they are in a state of 'deficiency'. One can express this as the following formula:

PERSON + DRUG = SUCCESS

where 'success' is defined as health, happiness, contentment, attractiveness, material success, fame or just adequate social functioning.

In this cultural atmosphere, many 'chemical comforters'—even pharmacologically active ones—are no longer perceived as 'drugs', and therefore attract less stigma. Jones (1979) found that although 80% of a group of patients agreed that heroin was a 'drug' only 50% classified morphine, sleeping tablets and tranquillizers as such, while only 33% saw aspirin as 'a drug'. In my own study of long-term users of benzodiazepines (Helman 1981) most users minimized the effect of the drug: 'Its not a drug—merely a thing for sleeping', 'It's a little bit of help—not a powerful drug'. Furthermore, there was evidence of having learnt and internalized an idealized model of behaviour, which could only be attained (or maintained) by the use of a drug. Without the psychotropic drug: 'I'd be miserable—take it out on the family', 'I couldn't help those I love', 'I'd be nervy, impatient with other people', 'If I didn't know of it [tranquillizer]—there would have been nothing I could do about it—I would think "I'm a miserable so-and-so and I'm stuck with it."' These attitudes are all expressions of a particular cultural milieu. It is one that is conducive both to the overuse of medications and to the effectiveness of placebos—especially if prescribed by a doctor or nurse.

THE CULTURAL CONSTRUCTION OF BELIEF

Much of the placebo effect is only part of a phenomenon known to anthropologists as *symbolic healing*—that is, all those forms of healing that do not rely on any physical or pharmacological treatments for their efficacy. They include the 'talk therapies' of Western psychology, such as psychotherapy and psychoanalysis, but also other forms of healing such as exorcisms, confession and counselling found in various religious, traditional and complementary therapies. As well as the use of certain ritual symbols in their 'microcontext', almost all involve healing through talk, action or various types of ritual. Often they aim at repairing relationships between people that have been damaged by illness or misfortune.

Most forms of 'symbolic healing' aim to be holistic: to have physical, psychological and social effects. However, one can differentiate between healing (emotional, cultural, social or spiritual change) and curing (change in physical state). Many traditional and religious healers make a pragmatic distinction between these two types of outcome (Csordas 1983). Their primary aim is to heal their clients emotionally, spiritually and even socially even if they cannot actually cure their physical disease.

Anthropologists such as Dow (1986) have tried to describe the universal features of all forms of symbolic healing: to understand how belief in a particular 'pill, potion or procedure' is actually created in the consultation. Dow identifies certain key stages in this process.

1. Healers (whether doctor, therapist, or traditional healer) must have some coherent system of explanation or frame of reference (that is, a cultural 'macrocontext') to explain the origin and nature of the problem, and how it can be dealt with. It may be one of germ theory or psychodynamic psychology, but may also be one of 'energy flow', 'witchcraft' or 'spirit possession'.

2. This frame of reference must include a symbolic bridge between personal experience, social relations and cultural meanings. That is, suffering people must be able to understand their own situation, and its resolution, in terms of its imagery, symbols and metaphors (as being due, say, to 'spirit possession', 'germ' invasion or 'intrapsychic conflict').

3. When patients consult healers, the healers aim to activate this symbolic bridge (that is, to convince clients—at least on the cognitive level—that their own particular problem can be explained and resolved in terms of the symbols of the frame of reference).

4. Once clients and healers have achieved this consensus, the healers need also to get patients emotionally—as well as intellectually—'attached' to the frame of reference: to link their hopes, fears, and anxieties to it. The patients have to become self-aware, and emotionally involved in the healing process itself. They need to be made to feel, for example, that their suffering is due to possession, by malevolent 'spirits', which if not treated could actually kill them.

5. Healers have then to guide therapeutic change by manipulating the symbols of their frame of reference. For example *curanderos*, having convinced clients that their symptoms are due to 'spirit possession', would

go through a ritual of exorcism. Afterwards they would tell them that the 'spirit' has left them—and they can now resume normal life as before. In this way, the clients learn to 'reframe' or reinterpret their recent experience in the light of the healer's frame of reference.

6. As well as being 'healed', clients have now acquired a new way of conceptualizing their experience in symbolic terms, and a new way of functioning. They have also acquired a new narrative: a new story that explains to them what has happened to them, and why, and how the healer was able to restore them to happiness or health.

This sequence of events—inherent in many placebo phenomena—applies as much in Harley Street as it does in the forests of New Guinea. In each case, the healer employs a variety of theatrical techniques, including the use of ritual symbols, as part of the healing process. These symbols derive from the local cultural context, and help to validate a particular frame of reference, and the healer that represents it.

THE NOCEBO EFFECT

Anthropologists have pointed out that belief can kill, as well as heal: that the placebo and nocebo effects are two sides of the same phenomenon (Hahn & Kleinman 1983). They have described many examples of the most extreme form of the nocebo effect, known as 'voodoo death' or 'hex death'. Although the exact physiological mechanism involved remains unknown (Lex 1977) a fuller understanding of the phenomenon depends on a knowledge of its context: of the beliefs, values, fears, anxieties and expectations of that community.

In 'voodoo death', a respected figure or healer in the tribe puts a public curse on an unfortunate individual, sometimes by 'pointing the bone'. Shortly afterwards that individual dies, apparently of natural causes. It has been reported in parts of Latin America, Africa, the Pacific, the Caribbean and amongst Australian Aborigines. The French anthropologist Levi-Strauss (1967) has described the atmosphere in such a case:

Shortly thereafter sacred rites are held to dispatch him to the realm of shadows. First brutally torn from all his family and social ties and excluded from all functions and activities through which he experienced self-awareness, then banished by the same forces from the world of the living, the victim yields to the combined terror, the sudden total withdrawal of the multiple reference systems provided by the support of the group, and finally to the group's decisive reversal in proclaiming him—once a living man, with rights and obligations—dead and an object of fear, ritual and taboo.

In this case, a form of *social death* precedes actual biological death. For that reason, Landy (1977) terms it 'socio cultural death'. Usually 'social death' (the community's ritual farewell to one of its members, at the funeral) follows biological death, after a variable period of time (Hertz 1960). In this case, however, the order is reversed. In that sense, it seems to be an example of what Engel (1971) termed the 'giving-up, given up' syndrome—which he saw as 'a life-setting conducive both to illness and to sudden death'. In his study of 170 unexplained sudden deaths, this syndrome was often a prelude to sudden death (usually without any physiological reason for this). For the individuals concerned, it was characterized by: (1) certain events that they could not ignore, (2) experience of overwhelming emotional excitation and (3) their belief that they have little or no control over the situation.

In the Western world, there are many other—though less extreme—opportunities for the nocebo effect. In each case, society regards such individuals as, in some form, 'socially dead' and withdraws social contact and support from them. In many cases this is likely to have some negative effect on their mental and physical health. These situations include: life imprisonment; long-term admission to a psychiatric hospital; and admission to an old-aged home, geriatric ward or home for the mentally handicapped. To some extent, certain medical diagnoses such as Alzheimer's disease, AIDS, certain types of disability or serious cancer may also have the same effect. In one study in the USA (Peters-Golden 1982), for example, 52% of a sample of women with breast cancer found that they were 'avoided' or 'feared', and only 3% felt that people were nicer to them than they had been before. Like other forms of the nocebo effect, this may be linked to deep-seated folk beliefs—such as seeing cancer as being due to 'demonic invasion' (Sontag 1978).

CONCLUSION

Any deeper understanding of both placebo and nocebo phenomena requires a knowledge of the *context*—physical, cultural, social and economic—in which they take place. This is because these contexts are absolutely intrinsic to the creation and maintenance of belief in the minds of both healer and patient, and all those around them.

REFERENCES

Campbell L V, Ashwell S M, Borkman M, Chisholm D 1992 White coat hyperglycaemia: disparity between diabetes clinic and home blood glucose concentrations. British Medical Journal 305:1194–1196
Claridge G 1970 Drugs and human behaviour. Allen Lane, London
Csordas T J 1983 The rhetoric of transformation in ritual healing. Medicine and Psychiatry 7:333–375
Dow J 1986 Universal aspects of symbolic healing: a theoretical synthesis. American Anthropologist 88
Editorial 1980 More anthropology and less sleep for medical students. British Medical Journal 281:1662
El-Islam M F 1982 Arabic cultural psychiatry. Transcultural Psychiatry Research Review 19:5–24

Engel G L 1971 Sudden and rapid death during psychological stress: folklore or folk wisdom? Annals of Internal Medicine 74:771–782

Hahn R A, Kleinman A 1983 Belief as pathogen, belief as medicine: 'voodoo death' and the 'placebo phenomenon' in anthropological perspective. Medical Anthropology Quarterly 14:3

Helman C G 1981 'Tonic', 'fuel' and 'food': social and symbolic aspects of the long-term use of psychotropic drugs. Social Science and Medicine 15B:521–533

Helman C G 2000 Culture, health and illness: an introduction for health professionals, 4th edn. Arnold, London, pp 1–11, 136–155

Hertz R 1960 Death and the right hand. Cohen and West, London, pp 27–86

Jones D R 1979 Drugs and prescribing: what the patient thinks. Journal of the Royal College of General Practitioners 29:417–419

Joyce C R B 1969 Quantitative estimates of dependence on the symbolic function of drugs. In: Steinberg H (ed) Scientific basis of drug dependence. Churchill Livingstone, New York, pp 271–280

Kleinman A 1978 The failure of Western medicine. Human Nature 1(11):63–68

Kleinman A 1980 Patients and healers in the context of culture. University of California Press, Berkeley, pp 312–319

Landy D (ed) 1977 Culture, disease and healing: studies in medical anthropology. Macmillan, New York, p 327

Levi-Strauss C 1967 Structural anthropology. Anchor, New York, pp 161–162

Lex B W 1977 Voodoo death: new thoughts on an old explanation. In: Landy D (ed) Disease, culture and healing: studies in medical anthropology. Macmillan, New York, pp 327–331

Long J, Gillilan R, Lee S G, Kim C R 1990 White-coat hypertension: detection and evaluation. Maryland Medical Journal 39:555–559

McDougall J 1989 Theatres of the body. Free Association, London, p 51

Martin M 1981 Native American medicine: thoughts for posttraditional healers. Journal of the American Medical Association 245:141–143

Mull J D 1983 A visit with a *curandero*. Western Journal of Medicine 139: 730–736

Pellegrino E D 1976 Prescribing and drug ingestion: symbols and substances. Drug Intelligence and Clinical Pharmacology 10:624–630

Peters-Golden H 1982 Breast cancer: varied perceptions of social support in illness experience. Social Science and Medicine 16:483–491

Rose L 1971 Faith healing. Penguin, Harmondsworth, p 54

Snow L F 1978 Sorcerer, saints and charlatans: black folk healers in urban America. Culture, Medicine and Psychiatry 2:69–106

Sontag S 1978 Illness as metaphor. Vintage, New York

Trethowan W H 1975 Pills for personal problems. British Medical Journal 3:749–751

Turner V W 1968 The drums of affliction. Clarendon, Oxford, pp 1–8

Turner V W 1969 The ritual process. Penguin, Harmondsworth, p 15

Warburton D M 1978 Poisoned people: internal pollution. Journal of Biosocial Science 10:309–319

Wolf S 1959 The pharmacology of placebos. Pharmacological Review ii: 689–705

2

Towards a scientific understanding of placebo effects

Edzard Ernst

Editor's note

Professor Ernzt reminds us that the term 'placebo response' includes and thereby confuses and obscures a host of ill-understood effects; effects that influence all forms of therapy to a greater or lesser degree. Improving certain aspects of the therapeutic encounter may enhance the outcome of *any* treatment, so Professor Ernzt encourages practitioners to learn about these elements and to use them well in everyday practice. He reminds us that the phrase so often used about complementary medicines, that they are 'just placebo', typifies the denial and misunderstanding of the many non-specific effects that contribute to self-healing responses and therapeutic outcomes. As science comes to understand consciousness and mind–body inter-relatedness better and can tease out the processes presently hidden in the black box we call 'placebo effects' the notion will almost certainly be abandoned.

The 'three stages of an artefact' seem to fit perfectly the historical development of the placebo effect: initially an 'artefact' is ignored, subsequently it is controlled for its presumed contaminating effects, then finally it is recognized and investigated as a phenomenon in its own right (Harrington 1997). Certainly placebo effects have been ignored and controlled (e.g. in controlled clinical trials). Only recently have we begun to realize their true importance and are directing systematic research towards it. Yet even today clinicians feel 'a shudder of discomfort like a cold hand in the dark' when considering that placebo effects are inevitably associated with whatever they do therapeutically (Wall 1992). Placebos are the ghosts that haunt the house of scientific objectivity, the creatures that rise up in the dark and expose the paradoxes and fissures in our definitions of the real and active factors in medical treatments (Ernst 1992). The 'aura of quackery' (Wall 1992) surrounding the placebo effect is, for many, too close for comfort. This holds true in particular for complementary medicine where therapists continuously are confronted with the sceptics' notion that their therapeutic successes are 'mere placebo effects'. Many myths that surround placebos seem to die hard (Ernst & Abbot 1996). The following is an attempt at demystifying the topic by assessing it scientifically and clarifying some of the confusion that often seems to surround the placebo effect.

WHAT ARE PLACEBO EFFECTS AND PLACEBOS?

Perhaps the earliest entry under placebo in a medical dictionary described placebo in 1785 as a treatment 'calculated to amuse for a time'. In a lexicon of 1811 a placebo is said to be 'given more to please than to benefit the patient' (Harrington 1997). A modern definition described placebo as 'any therapy or component of therapy that is used for its non-specific psychological or psychophysiological effect, or for its presumed specific effect, but is without specific activity for the condition being treated' (Shapiro & Morris 1978). This definition has its obvious problems— for instance, how do we define 'specific' and 'non-specific' effects? A more pragmatic definition may thus be called for (Gotzsche 1994): 'The placebo effect is the difference in outcome between a placebo treated group and an untreated control group in an unbiased experiment'. It reflects the impossibility of defining the placebo effect in a single case, where biases of various types cannot be excluded. A disarmingly simple definition was offered by Oh (1994): '[Placebo] … is the form of a treatment without its substance'. Unfortunately, this might not be applicable to all areas of medical treatment. At a NHI (National Health Institute) conference on the subject a 'consensus definition' was recently issued whereby a placebo effect is one that includes the many non-specific effects of therapy.

VARIOUS FACETS OF PLACEBO EFFECTS

Realizing the considerable difficulties in defining 'placebo', some have suggested that the concepts of placebos and placebo effects have outlived their usefulness altogether (Kirsch 1986, Omer & London 1989). One solution could be to use the terms 'placebo effects' synonymously with 'non-specific effects' and, in turn, differentiate these into various subunits, for example: 'physician attention; interest and concern in a healing setting; patient and physician expectations of treatment effects; the reputation, expense and impressiveness of the treatment; and characteristics of the setting that influence patients to report improvement' (Turner et al 1994). Each of these facets could then be researched in rigorously controlled experiments.

The 'perceived' placebo effect

The average response to the application of a placebo to a group of patients in a clinical trial is commonly equated with the placebo effect. This is not necessarily correct. Several other factors could also have played a role in bringing about this response (Ernst & Resch 1995a).

Natural course of the condition

Most diseases or symptoms will change over time. If, for example, the natural course of a condition investigated in a clinical trial (e.g. back pain or hypertension) were to decrease in time, this change would almost certainly exaggerate the perceived effect in the placebo arm of that study. Thus the natural history of such a condition can spuriously increase (or decrease) the perceived placebo effects in controlled clinical trials.

Most biological variables fluctuate. In situations where outcome measures are first measured when they are likely to be at or near a peak, a second measurement would probably give a lower reading. In other words, the blood pressure, pain or any other variable may, on average, be relatively high at entry and lower at the end of a treatment. This phenomenon is quite unrelated to effects of treatment or placebo. At first glance this phenomenon may seem unlikely, yet it can be very real indeed. Patients usually seek help because their complaint is at a peak. In clinical trials patients are often included because their symptom is present to a predefined degree (such as systolic blood pressure > 160 mmHg or pain at least moderate). In both cases a reading taken at a second visit would probably show that the outcome variable (e.g. blood pressure) had fallen, thus contributing substantially to the perceived placebo effect.

Investigator effects

To assume that the effect observed by administering a placebo for a given time (say 4 weeks) equals the placebo effect is to assume that all other factors influencing the outcome variable have remained constant. Yet several other factors exist that, depending on the clinical situation and setting, may change during this period of time. For example, the skill of the investigator in determining the outcome variable may have increased between the first and the last measurement. This in turn may lead to detection of larger (or smaller) pathological changes than before, which can thus decrease (or increase) the perceived placebo effect. There may also be time effects related to the patients. For example, 'white coat hypertension' (i.e. the fact that the mere presence of medical personnel raises a patient's blood pressure) would normally decrease as patients become used to the particular situation and environment. This, of course, would spuriously increase the perceived placebo effect in a trial of an antihypertensive therapy. There may also be seasonal and other time-dependent changes related to the outcome variable, which again could affect the size of the perceived placebo effect.

Changes in patients' behaviour

Once included in a trial, patients may become sensitized to the problem under investigation. Thus they might contribute, either deliberately or unconsciously, to the clinical outcome. Hypertensive patients could, for example, reduce their salt intake, try to avoid stress, or adopt other modifications of lifestyle simply because they are participating in a trial of an antihypertensive drug. Patients suffering from back pain may adapt their life to this new situation and therefore affect the clinical outcome. If not accounted for, these factors would tend to increase the size of the placebo effect as perceived in the placebo arm of a clinical trial.

(The influence of these and other confounding factors is considered in greater detail by Kienle & Kiene in Ch. 4.)

The 'true' placebo effect

The perceived placebo effect as seen in placebo-controlled trials is thus a function of several factors. It cannot be equated with the 'true' placebo effect (Ernst & Resch 1995a). In studies with a parallel untreated group (i.e. no placebo or other intervention, as with 'waiting list controls') these additional non-specific effects would produce the same response as in a placebo group (except for the true placebo effect). If one therefore subtracted the effects observed in such an untreated control group from those in the placebo group the 'true' placebo effect would be identified. Such 'three-armed' studies, it seems, are therefore the most unbiased way to investigate placebo effects in the setting of a clinical trial.

Further placebo-related terms

Pseudoplacebo

Pseudoplacebos are interventions that are active in principle but not for the condition that is being treated. They are widely used in clinical practice (e.g. a vitamin prescribed for a patient complaining about chronic insomnia) not least because they overcome some of the logistic and ethical problems of deliberate placebo use (e.g. the deception of the patient is perceived as less dishonest when an active drug is prescribed).

Superplacebo

Superplacebo is a term coined by the present author. It refers to a treatment that is, in fact, a placebo but neither the prescriber nor the patient is aware of the total lack of specific effects associated with it (Ernst 1992). Examples of superplacebos are treatments that were thought to work at the time they were used but were later found to be ineffective. Because all parties involved believed in them when they were prescribed, the placebo effect of superplacebos may be particularly powerful.

Hawthorne effect

The Hawthorne effect describes the tendency for people to change their behaviour because they are the target of special interest and attention. This may have the opposite direction to the placebo effect (Bouchet, Guillemin & Briacon 1996). The 'special interest or attention' could, for instance, be a diagnostic intervention.

Nocebo

Nocebo effects are adverse effects that can occur after the administration of placebos. They have characteristics much like side-effects of specific drugs. In controlled clinical trials, nocebo effects even tend to mimic the adverse effects of the active treatment given to the other treatment group.

CAN WE BE SURE THAT PLACEBO EFFECTS EXIST?

Perhaps surprisingly, some would answer this question with 'no' (Kienle 1995). A reanalysis of Beecher's classical paper (1955) suggested that the studies quoted by that author do not provide unequivocal proof of the existence of placebo effects. The placebo effects apparently observed in clinical trials could therefore be the result of a misattribution by patients of various naturally occurring and ambiguous changes in their clinical condition (Gibbon & Hormuth 1981, Ross & Olson 1981). In order to be sure that a 'perceived placebo effect' is a 'true placebo effect' an untreated control group is needed (see above). There are few studies that were conducted with both a placebo and an untreated control group (Ernst & Rasch 1995). A review of these trials shows that true placebo effects (of variable size) do exist beyond reasonable doubt. Thus both our clinical experience and scientific analysis of the available data confirm that placebo effects are real.

PLACEBO 'MYTHS'

Like few other medical subjects, placebo effects and placebos are surrounded by myths that are perpetuated in the literature. Here are some of them.

True and imagined illness

The opinion that one can differentiate between 'true' and 'imagined' disease by administering a placebo and observing who responds is widespread (e.g. Ernst & Abbot 1996) but cruelly wrong. The fact is that hypochondriacs, depressives, individuals with somatic pain and virtually all other types of patients can respond to placebo (Richardson 1989, Turner et al 1994, Wall 1992). To judge patients' credibility or trustworthiness on the basis of their placebo response would be a serious mistake and is often felt as a gross injustice by the patients concerned.

The placebo-responder personality

Another myth has it that a distinct placebo-responder personality exists. There has been a considerable amount of research on this topic; much of it has been contradictory. The best evidence, however, suggests that a responder personality cannot be differentiated from a non-responder personality. Absence of evidence is, however, not the same as evidence of absence. If a difference exists, and many clinicians carry on believing it does (Ernst & Abbot 1996), the nature of this difference has not yet been identified (Richardson 1994). A recent trial of homoeopathy inadvertently shed some light on this topic (Lepaisart 1995). In this study all patients were treated with placebo during a run-in phase and the 22% who showed a response to placebo were excluded from the trial proper. This was done with a view to excluding placebo responders from the subsequent experiment. In the trial phase that followed, one subgroup was treated with homoeopathic remedies and the other with placebo. In spite of previous placebo responders having been excluded, 75% of those receiving placebo during the second phase responded positively to it. Thus an individual who is a non-responder one day can become a responder the next or vice versa. No apparent reason seems to exist for this alteration in response.

(The placebo responder is discussed further by Philip Richardson in Ch. 3.)

Lack of quantifiable effect

Many clinicians assume that placebos affect only those parameters that cannot be quantified objectively. This is clearly wrong (Ernst 1992). On the contrary, the number and type of variables responsive to placebo seem to be limitless. Certainly objective and somatic variables are amongst them—even the concentration of constituents in patients' blood can be affected by placebos (e.g. Ernst 1992, Hashish, Feinman & Harvey 1988, Lepaisart 1995, Richardson 1994, Turner et al 1994). The fact that we know most of the placebo effects in pain does not exclude their existence elsewhere.

Beecher (1955) showed that in the 15 studies he reviewed an average of 35% of the patients responded to placebo. This led to the widespread misunderstanding that the size of the placebo effect is a constant of 35% (e.g. Lewith, Field & Machin 1983). The truth is that, depending on the exact details of the clinical situation, the placebo effect can vary from 0 to 100% (Liberman 1964, Richardson 1994).

Placebo treatment as 'doing nothing'

Many authors equate giving a placebo to patients with doing nothing at all (Ernst & Resch 1995b). This again is false. Most authors who equate placebos with no treatment probably do not want to make this point; quite simply, they are victims of confusion and sloppy thinking (Ernst & Resch 1995b). Yet this confusion is a reflection of a general attitude: 'this is *just* a placebo'. Few people seem to stop and think how useful placebos can actually be.

Degree and nature of placebo effect

A further myth has it that placebo effects are always mild. This may be true for most cases, yet as a generalization this notion does not hold true. The most dramatic example of this may be that of voodoo deaths (Ernst 1996, Harrington 1997). Theoretically, placebo effects can be stronger than the effects of active, demonstrably effective medication given for the same condition.

Many believe that placebo effects are necessarily positive—wrong again. Nocebo effects (i.e. adverse effects of placebos) can be demonstrated in the vast majority of placebo-controlled clinical trials. They may affect as many as 40% of patients taking placebos (Tangrea, Adrianza & Helsel 1994). In controlled trials, nocebo effects often mimic the nature of the side-effects of the active treatment (Cromie 1963). This most puzzling phenomenon could be due to (non-verbal?) communication, but at present it is far from being fully understood.

The most frequently reported nocebo effects are headache, drowsiness, tiredness, dizziness, nausea, pain and insomnia (Rosenzweis, Brochier & Zipfel 1993). This has to be seen against the fact that symptoms are also reported by healthy volunteers who take no medication at all; fatigue, headache and nasal congestion are the most frequent complaints in this situation (Meyer, Tröger & Röhl 1996).

Most controlled clinical trials obviously involve only short-term observations thus there is little research regarding the duration of placebo effects. The notion that placebo responses are necessarily short lived, however, seems to be wrong (Ross & Olsen 1982). More work is needed to clarify this issue.

Animal response

A final myth is that animals do not respond to placebos. Most people who care for pets will observe that animals respond to non-specific effects. Yet animals of course do not *know* they are receiving a medical intervention in the same way humans do. Pavlov's experiments are a good example of conditioning (see below) having physiological effects on animals.

HOW DO PLACEBOS WORK?

Having established that placebos do have effects, one might ask by what mechanisms these are brought about. A plethora of potential mechanisms of the placebo effect exist: operant conditioning, classical conditioning, guilt reduction, transference, suggestion, persuasion, role demands, hope, faith, labelling, selective symptom monitoring, misattribution, cognitive dissonance, control theory, anxiety reduction, expectancy effects, endorphin release and a variety of design and measurement artefacts (Richardson 1994). Most of these are based on little more than speculation. Some experimental evidence exists for the concepts of expectancy effects, cognitive dissonance, conditioning, anxiety reduction and endorphin release (Richardson 1994). Recent evidence suggests an inhibitory role of cholecystokinin in the placebo response, implying a more complex biology of placebo (Benedetti 1996). In each case, however, such findings are controversial. At present, therefore, the only conclusion that can be drawn is that the mode(s) of action of placebos is (are) not known.

WHICH FACTORS DETERMINE THE SIZE OF PLACEBO EFFECT?

Since the placebo response can vary from 0 to 100% (see above), it would be desirable to identify the factors that render one placebo more powerful than another. Once identified, one would try to make optimal use of these factors. This could make all types of medical treatments more effective without the risk of incurring costs or serious harm to patients. Thus, it would seem that this line of research is extremely relevant and potentially valuable. Several candidates for determinants exist, but to date they are largely speculative.

Nature of intervention

Surgery seems to be associated with extremely powerful placebo effects. The majority of patients submitted to 'sham-surgery' (skin incisions without an actual operation) show a response (Cobb et al 1959, Diamond, Kittle & Cockett 1960). Placebo injections provoke stronger reactions than placebo pills (Carne 1961, Grenfell, Briggs & Holland 1961). Invasiveness, discomfort or pain experienced by the patient is therefore likely to be an important factor in determining the size of the placebo effect. Similarly the colour (and size) of placebo pills partly determine the nature (and size) of the placebo effect (de Craen et al 1996). (see Ch. 12 for further details of this.)

The flavour of exoticism that surrounds therapies such as acupuncture or the magic of 'high tech' (e.g. ultrasound or laser therapy) or the unusual nature of a therapeutic encounter (e.g. history taking in homoeopathy or diagnostic procedures of traditional acupuncture) might all increase the placebo effect. It has been reported, for instance, that 100% of the patients treated with sham acupuncture respond positively (Taub et al 1979). Similarly interventions using sophisticated equipment (Langley & Sheppeard 1987, Schwitzgebel & Traugott 1968, Wickramasekera 1977) provoke an unexpectedly large placebo effect.

The therapist

Certain characteristics of the therapist induce stronger than average placebo responses. The status of professionals (Lesse 1962, Liberman 1961, Shapiro 1964), their confidence in the treatment (Uhlenhuth et al 1959), and the amount of empathy, warmth and understanding shown are some of the aspects that might play a role (Thomas 1987). The information transmitted to the patient about the disease could be another relevant determinant (Kaplan, Greenfield & Ware 1989). Intuitively one also feels that the therapist's expectations are of critical importance (Gracely et al 1985, Shapiro et al 1954). (The role of the therapist is discussed further in Ch. 3.)

The time factor

Although hard evidence is scarce, it seems conceivable that an extended patient/doctor interaction might lead to stronger placebo effects than a short encounter. The time factor might work indirectly by increasing trust, expectation, etc. On average, a patient's first consultation with a complementary practitioner lasts several times longer than one with a general practitioner (Fulder & Munro 1985, White, Resch & Ernst 1997).

Therefore sceptics have often argued that to a large extent this explains the therapeutic success of complementary therapists.

The patient

Patient expectation is probably one of the strongest determinants of the placebo response. It correlates positively with the observed outcome (e.g. Luparello et al 1970, Sternbach 1964). The general attitude of the patient towards the therapist is likely to exert a similar influence. Trust, it seems, is an important prerequisite for a powerful placebo effect. Patient involvement with the therapy could be another factor. The administration of a topical placebo involving patients in their treatment has been shown to lead to more powerful effects than does the oral administration of placebo (Saradeth, Resch & Ernst 1994).

The nature of the complaint

Some conditions might respond better to placebo than others. Much of the research on placebo has been conducted in conditions associated with pain. We know that most other complaints and symptoms also respond to placebo (Ernst & Resch 1995a). It would be valuable to readdress the question in a systematic way to determine whether some conditions or diseases are inherently more 'placebo prone' than others.

The therapeutic setting

In a recent study, the therapeutic setting was the only significant predictor for nocebo effects (Tangrea, Adrianza & Helsel 1994). The authors were unable to determine more precisely what the important characteristics of the setting were. Intuitively one might think, for instance, that a formal clinical setting is more effective than an informal one.

THE 'PHARMACOLOGY' OF PLACEBOS

Placebo effects have characteristics that are strikingly similar to those of active medication. A dose–effect relationship (Blackwell, Bloomfield & Buncher 1972), time–effect curves, cumulated effects after repeated administration and carry-over effects after cessation of placebo administration have all been described (Lasagna, Laties & Dohan 1958). Placebos can also have complex interactions with other (active) medication (Kleijen et al 1994).

As pointed out above, placebos can lead to unwanted side-effects. They can also produce worsening of symptoms (Shapiro, Wilensky & Struening 1968); even cases of 'placebo dependence' have been described (Boleloucky 1971, Vinar 1969).

PLACEBOS IN CLINICAL PRACTICE

The majority of healthcare professionals do have experience with the deliberate use of placebos (Ernst & Abbot 1996, Goodwin, Goodwin & Voger 1979, Gray & Flynn 1981). Yet in official, routine healthcare placebo treatments have remained somewhat of a taboo (Wall 1992). Using placebos outside of clinical trials has an aftertaste of charlatanism—not least because it involves deceiving the patient. Therefore some feel that deliberate placebo administration is unethical. In complementary medicine the often-heard phrase 'this is just a placebo' contributes crucially to a climate of denial and misunderstanding of placebo effects.

Even if one is opposed to prescribing a dummy pill in clinical practice, one might be well advised to maximize the placebo effect that is associated with (almost any) specific therapy. Whenever we treat patients, the placebo effect is part of the therapeutic response. Depending on the particular situation, one might be able to optimize the placebo response by emphasizing and using one or more of its potential determinants (see above) during the therapeutic encounter. For instance, empathic reassurance will produce better results than truth and uncertainty (Uhlenhuth et al 1959). It would follow that the optimal therapy is to use (where possible) an active therapy plus all the features that provoke a powerful placebo response.

CONCLUSION

Until recently, the history of medicine was a history of placebo. Pharmacopoeias of all origins were full with placebos without physicians realizing it. Thus the placebo effect was largely ignored. After highly effective treatments had become available, placebos were predominantly used in clinical trials. Thus the placebo effect was being controlled. Only recently have we entered the 'third stage of an artefact' (Harrington 1997) and begun to appreciate the placebo effect in its own right. If we want to optimize (rather than ignore or control) the placebo effect, we need to understand it better than we do today. To reach this aim we should discard several persistent myths and investigate in detail the determinants of its power.

REFERENCES

Beecher H K 1955 The powerful placebo. Journal of the Americal Medical Association 159:1602–1606
Benedetti F 1996 The opposite effects of the opiate antagonist naloxone and the acholecystokinin antagonist proglumide on placebo analgesia. Pain 64:535–543.
Blackwell B, Bloomfield S S, Buncher C R 1972 Demonstration to medical students of placebo responses and non-drug factors. Lancet 1:1279–1282
Boleloucky Z 1971 A contribution to the problems of placebo dependence: a case report. Activitas Nervosa Superior 13:190–191

Bouchet C, Guillemin C, Briacon S 1996 Non-specific effects in longitudinal studies. Impact on quality of life measurements. Journal of Clinical Epidemiology 49:15–20

Carne S 1961 The action of chorionic gonadotrophin in the obese. Lancet ii:1282–1284

Cobb L A, Thomas G I, Dillard D H et al 1959 An evaluation of internal mammary artery ligation by a double blind technique. New England Journal of Medicine 260:1115–1118

Cromie B W 1963 The feet of clay of the double blind trial. Lancet 9:994–997

de Craen A J M, Roos P J, de Vries A L, Kleijnen J 1996 Effect of colour of drugs: systematic review of perceived effect of drugs and their effectiveness. British Medical Journal 313:1624–1626

Dimond E G, Kittle C F, Cockett J E 1960 Comparison of internal mammary artery ligation and sham operation for angina pectoris. Americal Journal of Cardiology 4:483–486

Ernst E 1992 Placebo forte. Wiener Medizinische Wochenschrift 142:217–219

Ernst E 1996 Make believe medicine. The amazing powers of placebo. European Journal of Physical Medicine and Rehabilitation 6(4):124–125

Ernst E, Abbot N C 1996 Placebos in clinical practice, results of a survey of nurses. Perfusion 4:128–130

Ernst E, Resch K-L 1995a The concept of the perceived and true placebo effect. British Medical Journal 311:551–553

Ernst E, Resch K-L 1995b The importance of placebo effects. Journal of the American Medical Association 273:283

Fulder S J, Munro R E 1985 Complementary medicine in the United Kingdom: patients, practitioners and consultations. Lancet 1985:542–545

Gibbon S F, Hormuth S E 1981 Motivational factors in placebo responsivity. Psychopharmacology Bulletin 17:77–79

Goodwin J S, Goodwin J M, Voger A V 1979 Knowledge and use of placebo by house officers and nurses. Annals of Internal Medicine 91:106–110

Gotzsche P 1994 Is there logic in the placebo? Lancet 344:925–926

Gracely R H, Dubner R, Deeter W R et al 1985 Clinicians' expectations influence placebo analgesia. Lancet 1:43

Gray G, Flynn P 1981 A survey of placebo use in general hospital. General Hospital Psychiatry 3:199–203

Grenfell R, Briggs A H, Holland W C 1961 A double-blind study of the treatment of hypertension. Journal of the American Medical Association 176:124–167

Harrington A 1997 The placebo effect. Harvard University Press, Cambridge, M A

Hashish I, Feinman C, Harvey W 1988 Reduction of postoperative pain and swelling by ultrasound: a placebo effect. Pain 83:303–311

Kaplan S H, Greenfield S, Ware J E 1989 Assessing the effects of physician–patient interactions on the outcomes of chronic disease. Medical Care 27(suppl):110–127

Kienle G S 1995 Der sogenannte Placeboeffekt. Illusion, Fakten, Realität. Schattaner, Stuttgart

Kirsch I 1986 Unsuccessful redefinitions of the term placebo. American Journal of Psychology 41:844–845

Kleijnen J, de Craen A J M, van Everdingen J et al 1994 Placebo effect in double-blind clinical trials: a review of interactions with medications. Lancet: 344:1347–1349

Langley G B, Sheppeard H 1987 Transcutaneous electrical nerve stimulation (TNS) and its relationship to placebo therapy: a review. New Zealand Medical Journal 100:215–217

Lasagna L, Laties V G, Dohan J L 1958 Further studies on the 'pharmacology' of placebo administration. Journal of Clinical Investigation 37:533–537

Lepaisart C 1995 Clinical trials in homeopathy: treatment of mastodynia due to premenstrual syndrome. Revue Francaise de Gynecologie et d'Obstetrique 90:94–97

Lesse S 1962 Placebo reactions in psychotherapy. Diseases of the Nervous System 12:313–319

Lewith G T, Field J, Machin D 1983 Acupuncture compared with placebo in post herpetic pain. Pain 16:361–368

Liberman R 1961 Analysis of the placebo phenomenon. Journal of Chronic Diseases 15:761–783

Liberman R 1964 An experimental study of the placebo response under three different situations of pain. Journal of Psychiatric Research 2:233–246

Luparello T, Leist N, Lourie C H et al 1970 The interaction of psychologic stimuli and pharmacologic agents on airway reactivity in asthmatic subjects. Psychosomatic Medicine 32:509–513

Meyer F P, Tröger U, Röhl F-W 1996 Adverse non-drug reactions, an update. Clinical Pharmacology and Therapeutics 60:347–352

Oh V M 1994 The placebo effect: can we use it better? British Medical Journal 309:69–70

Omer H, London P 1989 Signal and noise in psychotherapy: the role and control of nonspecific factors. British Journal of Psychiatry 155:239–245

Richardson P H 1989 Placebos: their effectiveness and modes of action. In: Broome A (ed) Health psychology: processes and applications. Chapman & Hall, London, pp 35–56

Richardson P H 1994 Placebo effects in pain management. Pain Reviews 1:15–32

Rosenzweig P, Brochier S, Zipfel A 1993 The placebo effect in healthy volunteers: influence of experimental conditions on the adverse events profile during phase I studies. Clinical Pharmacology and Therapeutics 54:578–583

Ross M, Olson J M 1981 An expectancy attribution model of the effects of placebos. Psychological Review 81:408–437

Ross M, Olson J M 1982 Placebo effects in medical research and practice. In: Eiser J R (ed) Social psychology and behavioural medicine. Wiley, Chichester, pp 441–458

Saradeth T, Resch K-L, Ernst E 1994 Placebo for varicose veins—don't eat it, rub it! Phlebology 9:63–66

Schwitzgebel R, Traugott M 1968 Initial note on the placebo effect of machines. Behavioural Medicine 13:267–273

Shapiro A K 1964 Etiological factors in placebo effect. Journal of the American Medical Association 187:712–714

Shapiro A K, Morris L A 1978 The placebo effect in medical and psychological therapies. In: Bergin A E, Garfield S (eds) Handbook of psychotherapy and behavioural change. John Wiley, New York, pp 369–410

Shapiro A K, Wilensky H, Struening E L 1968 Study of the placebo effect with a placebo test. Comprehensive Psychiatry 9:118–137

Shapiro A P, Myers T, Reiser M F et al 1954 Comparison of blood pressure response to Veriloid and to the doctor. Psychosomatic Medicine 16:478–488

Sternbach R A 1964 The effects of instructional sets on autonomic responsivity. Psychophysiology 1:67–72

Tangrea J A, Adrianza E, Helsel W E 1994 Risk factors for the development of placebo adverse reactions in a multicenter clinical trial. Annals of Epidemiology 4:327–331

Taub H A, Mitchell J N, Stuber F E, Eisenberg L, Beard M C, McCormack R K 1979 Analgesia for operative dentistry: a comparison of acupuncture and placebo. Oral Surgery 48(3):205–210

Thomas K B 1987 General practice consultations: is there any point in being positive? British Medical Journal 294:1200–1202

Turner J A, Deyo R A, Loeser J D et al 1994 The importance of placebo effects in pain treatment and research. Journal of the American Medical Association 271:1609–1614

Uhlenhuth E H, Canter A, Neustadt J O et al 1959 The symptomatic relief of anxiety with meprobamate, phenobarbital and placebo. American Journal of Psychiatry 115:905–910

Vinar O 1969 Dependence on a placebo: a case report. British Journal of Psychiatry 115:1189–1190

Wall P D 1992 The placebo effect, an unpopular topic. Pain 51:1–3

White A R, Resch K-L, Ernst E 1997 A survey of complementary practitioners' fees, practice, and attitudes to working within the National Health Service. Complementary Therapies in Medicine 5:210–214

Wickramasekera I 1977 The placebo effect and medical instruments and biofeed-back. Journal of Clinical Engineering 2:227–230

3

A critical reanalysis of the concept, magnitude and existence of placebo effects

Gunver S. Kienle and Helmut Kiene

Editor's note

Having so long emphasised technical effectiveness, modern medicine is beginning to understand just how important as yet poorly defined human factors can be. As practitioners we usually take our clinical impressions of treatment outcomes as the measure of our effectiveness. Yet though we say these everyday experiences justify the way we treat patients, our results may have less to do with specific treatments than with these non-specific factors. Calling them 'placebo effect' just creates a rag-bag category; nor is labelling something the same as understanding it - or how it works. For nearly 50 years since Beecher's classic research, the myth of the 30% placebo response has persisted. Dr Kienle takes it apart and criticises subsequent studies that appear to show even higher rates of placebo response. In doing this she highlights many of the non-specific factors that influence treatment outcome, and asks whether the placebo response (in its narrow sense of mere imitation therapy) exists at all. By re-examining these studies she has been able to identify in every case, significant non-pharmacological factors at work. Her chapter makes us more aware of what they might be. She introduces the term 'patient self-healing' and implies that it is right and proper for practitioners to encourage these processes.

Since 1955, when H. K. Beecher published his classic 'The powerful placebo', it has been generally accepted that 35% of patients with any of a wide variety of disorders can be treated with placebos alone. In recent years average cure rates of 70%, and up to 100%, also have been quoted. However, in recent analyses the source material that forms the scientific basis for such claims has been examined. These analyses show that the studies on which such ideas had been based, except perhaps in bronchial asthma, do not in any way justify the conclusions drawn from them. The truth is that the placebo effect is counterfeited by a variety of factors including the natural history of the disease, regression to the mean, concomitant treatments, obliging reports, experimental subordination, severe methodological defects in the studies, misquotations, etc.—even, on occasion, by the fact that the supposed placebo is actually not a placebo but has to be acknowledged as having a specific action on the condition for which it is being given. A further reason for misjudgement is the lack of clarity of the placebo concept itself. The placebo topic seems to invite negligent methodological and conceptual thinking. Our conclusion in this chapter is that the literature relating to the magnitude and frequency of the placebo effect is unfounded and grossly overrated, if not entirely false. We also pose the question of whether the existence of the so-called placebo effect is itself not largely—or indeed totally—illusory.

AN ANALYSIS OF RESEARCH FINDINGS

'The study of the placebo is the most important step to be taken in scientific therapy' (Conferences on therapy 1946). With these words, the scientific study of the placebo effect was inaugurated. Nine years later, H. K. Beecher (1955) published his sensational and pioneering article, 'The powerful placebo', in which the magnitude of the placebo effect was first quantitated. On the basis of 15 studies Beecher concluded that, in a number of different diseases, 35% of patients could be adequately treated by the administration of placebo alone. Since Beecher's article was published, the therapeutic placebo effect seems to have been elevated to the level of scientific fact.

The number of publications on the placebo effect has since grown to almost boundless proportions, though 'The powerful placebo' still remains the most important and most frequently cited reference work in this area (Bodem 1994, Moerman 1983, Roberts 1995, Turner et al 1994). Since Beecher's study, descriptions of therapeutic placebo effects have been extended to virtually every variety of disease. The magnitude of the placebo effect is often no longer given as 35%, as Beecher suggested, but as 70%, or even as high as 100%. Scepticism aroused by such high placebo response rates has led the authors of the present article to carry out a thorough reanalysis of a large number of publications on which these rates are based (Kienle 1995, Kienle & Kiene 1996, 1997).

First, Beecher's article was reanalysed, with surprising results (Kienle 1995, Kienle & Kiene 1997). In contrast to his claim, no evidence was found of any placebo effect in any of the studies cited by him. There were many methodological mistakes that severely flawed the interpretation. Many other factors were found that could account for the reported improvements in patients in these trials, but most likely there was no placebo effect whatsoever.

When further often-cited and well-known placebo trials and placebo surveys (Bodem 1994, Ernst & Resch 1995, Moerman 1983, Netter, Classen & Feingold 1986, Roberts et al 1993, Turner et al 1994) were reanalysed (Kienle 1995, Kienle & Kiene 1996)—altogether 800 articles—the results were the same again: the publications displayed similar mistakes and, with great plausibility, did not demonstrate any therapeutic placebo effects (Kienle 1995, Kienle & Kiene 1996, 1997).

Many factors and mistakes were found that create illusions of thera-peutic placebo effects; they are summarized in Box 4.1. The distribution of these mistakes in Beecher's 'The powerful placebo' is shown in Table 4.1. These factors are still prevalent in modern placebo literature. Thus, aware-ness of Beecher's mistakes and misinterpretations is essential for an appro-priate interpretation of current placebo literature. In the following several examples will be presented, most of which are taken from Beecher (1955) and from other classical or important placebo surveys (Bodem 1994, Ernst & Resch 1995, Meyer & Kindli 1989, Moerman 1983, Netter, Classen & Feingold 1986, Turner et al 1994).

Box 4.1 Factors that can cause the false impression of a placebo effect (Kienle 1995, Kienle & Kiene 1997)

- Natural course of a disease:
  — spontaneous improvement
  — fluctuation of symptoms
  — regression to the mean
- Additional treatment
- Observer bias:
  — conditional switching of treatment
  — scaling bias
- Irrelevant response variables
- Patient bias:
  — polite answers and experimental subordination
  — conditioned answers
  — neurotic or psychotic misjudgement
- No placebo given at all:
  — psychotherapy
  — psychosomatic phenomena
  — voodoo medicine
- The placebo is not a placebo
- Uncritical reporting of anecdotes
- Misquotation
- False assumption of toxic placebo effects created by:
  — everyday symptoms
  — misquotation
  — persistence of symptoms

Table 4.1 Factors that created the illusion of a placebo effect in H. K. Beecher's study list (Kienle 1995, Kienle & Kiene 1997)

Study	a	b	c	d	e	f	g	h	i	j	k	l	m	n	o
% of patients that were 'satisfactorily relieved by a placebo', according to Beecher (Netter, Classen & Feingold 1986)	35	38	52	58	26	38	21	26	31	37	26–40	30	15–53	36–43	30
Factors creating illusions of placebo effect															
Spontaneous improvement	x	x		x	x		x	x	x			x	x	x	
Spontaneous fluctuation of symptoms		x		x	x		x				x				
Conditional switching of treatment	x	x			x			x	x	x					
Scaling bias	x	x			x										
Additional treatment	x			x											
Irrelevant response variables				x	x										x
Polite answers									x	x		x			
Conditioned answers									x	x		x			
Neurotic or psychotic misjudgement											x				
Misquotation			x	x		x		x	x	x	x	x	x	x	
Everyday symptoms misinterpreted as placebo side-effects												x			x
Habituation			x						x						
Poor definition of drug efficacy				x	x										x
Subsiding toxic effect of previous medication							x								x
Demonstration of a placebo effect?	no	no	/*	no	no	no	no	no	no	no	no	no	no	no	no

Studies: [a]Diehl 1933, [b]Evans & Hoyle 1933, [c]Jellinek 1946, [d]Gay & Carliner 1949, [e]Travell et al 1949, [f]Greiner et al 1950, [g]Keats & Beecher 1950, [h]Keats, Alessandro & Beecher 1951, [i]Beecher et al 1951, [j]Hillis 1952, [k]Beecher et al 1953, [l]Wolf & Pinsky 1954, [m]Lasagna et al 1954, [n]Gravenstein, Devloo & Beecher 1954, [o]Lasagna, Felsinger & Beecher 1955.
*The publication (Jellinek 1946) gives no account of the study design.

THE DILEMMA OF THE PLACEBO CONCEPT

When approaching the topic of placebos, one is first confronted with a wide variety of usages of the terms 'placebo' and 'placebo effect'. Beecher (1955) defined placebos as 'pharmacologically inert substances'. Still today, a similar description is given: 'A placebo is a pharmacologically inactive substance that can have a therapeutic effect if administered to a patient who believes that he or she is receiving an effective treatment' (Iacono et al 1992). However, broader formulations of the concept also exist.

From the pharmacological viewpoint, it might be useful to distinguish between *pharmacological* and *non-pharmacological* therapies, and to apply a global label of 'placebo' to the latter. This extends the concept of placebo to all forms of psychotherapy, creative therapy and psychological healing effects, as well as to all forms of drug therapy that do not have a recognized pharmacological basis. Still, this conclusion is beset with problems—in fact, it is incorrect. It assumes, first of all, that the mere administration of inert imitation drugs can be as successful as those forms of therapy mentioned above—an assumption that first should be subjected to accurate testing. Secondly, these therapies (unlike the administration of imitation drugs) are characterized by claims to their own active principles, and by differentiated and professionalized matching of diagnoses and treatments.

In general, attempts are made to subdivide placebo and non-placebo treatments on the basis of a *specificity/non-specificity* dichotomy; however, this also appears to have failed (Kienle & Kiene 1996). The verdict was finally articulated by Gøtzsche (1994): 'In conclusion, the placebo concept as presently used cannot be defined in a logically consistent way and leads to contradictions.'

There follow three main reasons why the concept of the placebo *cannot* be defined conclusively in terms of the notion of the non-specific (e.g. non-specific activity, non-specific effect, not containing a specific ingredient, etc.).

1. In general, any definition is subject to Albert's trilemma so that, in principle, definitions cannot be formulated in a consistent way (Albert 1991, Kienle 1995).

2. The concept of the non-specific introduces additional problems. Something that is non-specific (or indeterminate) cannot be positively determined as being so, but can only be negatively determined by exclusion of what is specific in the case in question.

3. In the case of a therapy, in order to exclude the specific components it is necessary to know *all* the specific modes of action. At best, however, scientists can know only those modes of action that already have been discovered and are already known to them as such. Consequently, there can never be any certainty that all specific modes of action have been excluded.

How difficult it is in practice to exclude specific therapeutic principles can be demonstrated by a more detailed examination of the situational context in which drug administration takes place. (The effects of the situational context often are classified as non-specific or placebo effects.) This is a context in which the doctor and patient meet on both verbal and non-verbal levels, but neither the verbal nor the non-verbal level can be classed as entirely non-specific. For example, on the verbal level, a patient with intermediate-grade myocardial failure may be advised to restrict fluid and salt intake and to avoid swimming. If this verbal advice is followed, it leads to the adoption of measures that specifically are beneficial to the health or the very survival of the patient in heart failure.

In a similar way, specific effects also can be achieved on the non-verbal level. For example, randomized double-blind studies have yielded good evidence that prayer by uninvolved persons can exert a statistically significant beneficial effect on the course of a patient's illness (Byrd 1988, Dossey & Schellhorn 1995). Dossey & Schellhorn point out that such effects are *not* placebo effects, but that they are specifically brought about by the prayer. This contention, after all, is supported by the fact that these effects were demonstrated in a double-blind study. Although such findings may appear eccentric, they nevertheless demonstrate the possibility that within the therapeutic encounter a particular internal attitude on the part of the physician may lead to therapeutic efficacy in the patient—which, as Dossey says, is *not* a non-specific effect. These examples should suffice to demonstrate that, in the encounter between physician and patient, it is difficult to draw a line between the specific and non-specific components of therapy.

Ultimately, then, it is impossible to define what a placebo is. None the less, Hornung (1994) has cut this gordian knot. He defined a placebo as an inert preparation that looks like an active medication. Whether something is an inert preparation, says Hornung, can be agreed on in each individual case. This pragmatic solution is ultimately acceptable. For the purposes of our following presentation, however, it must be borne in mind that the term 'placebo' will be applied only to the *imitation* of a treatment, and not to all those therapeutic endeavours aimed at mobilizing the body's self-healing powers. (Whether these psychotherapeutic, creative-therapeutic or similar endeavours are more effective than the mere administration of a placebo is a question that is not the focus of the present article.)

Regardless of the uncertainties of the placebo *concept*, the placebo *effect* can be defined as the 'therapeutic effect of a placebo administration'. Box 3.2 shows criteria through which such therapeutic placebo effects can be assessed. As will be shown further on, illusions of the existence of such effects can be produced by many factors.

FACTORS THAT CAN CREATE FALSE IMPRESSIONS OF PLACEBO EFFECTS

Natural, spontaneous improvement of a disease

'Sick people often get better' (Liberman 1962)—this simple fact often seems to be forgotten in placebo literature. Yet it is evident that the natural course of a disease is not an effect of any drug administration; it is an improvement that occurs spontaneously, irrespective of any therapeutic interventions.

Box 4.2 Hierarchical criteria for the assessment of clinical and experimental studies in relation to the question of whether a therapeutic placebo effect has been convincingly documented (Kienle & Kiene 1996)*

I. Basic criteria
1. Was a placebo *actually given* in the investigation?
2. Does the study fulfil the *minimal methodological criteria*: correct quotation of data; comprehensible and convincing description in the publication; no patient selection; reasonable outcome measures; consistent patient treatment; etc.?
3. Was a *therapeutically relevant outcome measure* selected for the study? (The measure may be experimentally generated, but must then correspond to a disease or a disease-related symptom.)

II. Efficacy criteria
4. Does the investigation demonstrate a *change in the outcome measures* on placebo treatment?
5. Is this change in the outcome measures an *effect of placebo administration* (or was it counterfeited by other factors, e.g. natural variation in the disease, regression to the mean, simultaneous or prior therapy, etc.)?
6. Is the effect of placebo administration a *true effect* (or only a verbal effect, obliging report, or an instance of experimental subordination)?

III. Clinical criterion
7. Was cure of a disease or improvement in disease-related symptomatology (not experimentally produced symptoms) investigated in the study?

* If a study satisfies all the basic criteria (1–3), it can be used in considering the question of placebo efficacy; if a study additionally satisfies all the efficacy criteria (4–6), a *true* placebo effect has been demonstrated; if a study additionally satisfies the clinical criterion (7), a true *therapeutic* placebo effect has been demonstrated.

Very often, however, in placebo literature the spontaneous improvement of a disease is falsely named a placebo effect. For instance, in a placebo-controlled drug trial on acute common cold described as mild and of short duration, 35% of the patients felt better within 2–6 days (Diehl 1933). Beecher (1955) interpreted these improvements as an effect of the placebo administration. However, he did not consider that many patients with a mild common cold improve spontaneously within 6 days (as already pointed out in the original publication (Diehl 1933)).

Other trials reported by Beecher concern postoperative pain (Beecher et al 1953, Keats & Beecher 1950, Keats, D'Alessandro & Beecher 1951, Lasagna et al 1954). It is a characteristic feature of postoperative pain that it diminishes naturally during the days following the operation. From data in the original publications of these trials (Kienle 1995) one can see that the supposed therapeutic placebo effect was of the same magnitude as the spontaneous diminishing of postoperative pain. Again, the spontaneous improvement has been mistaken as a placebo effect. For the same mistake, numerous other trials (including recent ones) could be referred to.

Spontaneous fluctuation of symptoms or disease course

In chronic diseases fluctuation of symptoms or of the course of disease should be taken into account. Patients feel better one day and worse the next. Therefore, looking at a number of chronically ill patients one will simply always see some patients improving. Because of this, it is a mistake to ignore the rate of deterioration and only report the rate of improvement and call the latter a placebo 'effect'. This fallacy is rather frequent in placebo trials. Some examples follow.

• It was claimed that 20% of patients with *angina pectoris* were successfully treated by placebo (Meyer & Kindli 1989, Netter, Classen & Feingold 1986). In fact, in the placebo group 20% of the patients got better; however 72% got worse (LeRoy 1941).

• A 56% placebo effect was claimed in patients with *irritable colon* because half of the placebo group improved (Meyer & Kindli 1989, Netter, Classen & Feingold 1986). However, it was not mentioned that the other half got worse (Lichstein, DeCosta Mayer & Hauch 1955). Additionally, patients were put on a special diet.

• A 21% placebo effect was claimed in the treatment of a *cerebral infarction*, because 21% of the patients in the placebo group improved (Meyer & Kindli 1989, Netter, Classen & Feingold 1986). However, it was not mentioned that 53% of the patients died. Of course neither the improvement of 21% nor the death of 53% of patients can be attributed to the placebo administration. Besides, every patient got the best medical and physiotherapeutic care available (Dyken & White 1956).

• Another example is a study of *chronic pain* that also fluctuated spontaneously (Deyo 1993, Whitney & Von Korff 1992). There was pain relief in 13% and a deterioration in 20% of the patients given placebo. According to the author's interpretation the 13% improvement was caused by the therapeutic power of the placebo, whereas the 20% impairment was caused by the toxic power of placebo (Long, Uematsu & Kouba 1989). Again the spontaneous fluctuation was not taken into account.

Many more examples could be given.

Regression to the mean

Both fluctuation of symptoms or disease course and natural improvement of a disease are special forms of a regression to the mean, which always has to be considered when observations are started with values strongly deviating from the norm. In this situation subsequent observations are statistically more likely to measure more relatively normal ('improved') values than to measure more extreme values. It is in the latter circumstances that patients tend to consult physicians, because patients generally look for medical help when their symptoms are at a peak (Whitney & Von Korff 1992). In these situations symptoms will statistically improve rather than deteriorate. In their interesting article, 'How much of the placebo "effect" is really statistical regression?' McDonald, Mazzuca & McCabe (1983) have argued that 'most improvements attributed to the placebo effect are actually instances of statistical regression'.

Additional treatment

In many trials that supposedly demonstrate placebo effectiveness the patients received additional effective treatment. Examples concerning irritable colon and cerebral infarction have already been mentioned. For instance, in a trial referred to by Beecher (1955), patients with angina pectoris were given placebos *plus* nitrates (Travell et al 1949). Another example is the survey by Moerman (1983) concerning placebo-controlled cimetidin trials in gastric and duodenal ulceration. As 10 to 90% of patients in placebo groups improved, a 10–90% placebo effectiveness has been claimed (Moerman 1983, Turner et al 1994). However, additional treatment and support was not taken into account: the improvement rates were dependent on hospitalization (stress reduction), length of observation, smoking habits of the patients, and advice concerning diet, nicotine, alcohol and drugs; besides which, patients were also given antacids.

Conditional switching of treatment

In one trial referred to by Beecher (1955), the patients with angina pectoris were treated in the following manner: as long as the patients had only minor complaints, they were treated with placebos, but when anginal episodes increased, they were switched to the test drug. Thus, good periods were selected for placebo treatment, and bad periods were selected for drug treatment (Evans & Hoyle 1933). Similarly, in two other trials that Beecher (1955) referred to, patients were excluded from evaluation when their condition deteriorated and they were included again as soon as they had improved (Beecher et al 1951, 1953)—of course, this kind of patient selection creates the illusion of effective placebo therapies.

Irrelevant or questionable response variables

Immense placebo effects can be claimed when they are based on response variables that are irrelevant for the condition in question (Kienle 1995). For instance, there is a claim of a 73% placebo effect in multiple sclerosis (Netter, Classen & Feingold 1986). However, the facts in the original publication (Blomberg 1957) were that no objective change in the neurological condition was found in any patient on placebo, yet 73% of the patients had the subjective feeling of increased euphoria, strength and agility. However, euphoria is itself a symptom of multiple sclerosis; therefore an increase of euphoria is not necessarily a sign of improvement. Spontaneous variation of euphoric and optimistic answers is typical for this disease and therefore these are inappropriate response variables for demonstrating placebo effects.

Another claim is a 62% placebo effect in hypertension (Netter, Classen & Feingold 1986). The facts in the original trial (Coe, Best & Kinsman) were that there was no significant change in blood pressure under placebo, but 61% of the patients subjectively felt better. However, all patients had first received veratrum, which caused severe toxic symptoms in 64% of the patients. It was then substituted by placebos. Therefore the relief of symptoms in 61% of placebo-treated patients can be explained by the cessation of veratrum toxicity (Kienle 1995). There is no reason to assume any placebo effect in this case.

Answer of politeness and experimental subordination

Polite answers and experimental subordination are key problems in judging placebo effects, but they are hardly ever considered in the placebo literature. 'Polite answer' means that patients report improvement just to please the doctor, whereas in fact nothing has improved. Roberts (1995) describes it as follows: 'The word "placebo" means "to please" but this applies to both the patient and the doctor. For example, patients may report positive outcomes to their physicians out of a need to "be polite" to them.' The problem has been characterized by Sackett (1995): 'Finally, when the patient is grateful for clinician's time and effort in trying to help them, this gratitude (plus simple good manners) often is reflected in an exaggeration of the benefits of the latest prescription when they are asked "Did that medicine help you?"'

A similar phenomenon is what is called 'experimental subordination' (Kiene 1993, 1996a, b). This means that in an experiment subjects say what they think is expected of them, rather than what they really experience. This phenomenon has been described by several authors (Barber 1963, Clark 1969, Fordyce et al 1984, Tedeschi, Schenkler & Bonoma 1971).

It is not always easy to avoid such patient bias. Nevertheless it is a key point in placebo research (Kienle & Kiene 1996), since it is easier to provoke some effect within the answers of the patient than within the real disease of the patient. Of course, a polite answer or an experimental subordination is not a placebo effect itself but the mere *illusion* of a placebo effect.

Conditioned answers

It seems difficult to differentiate therapeutic placebo effects from conditioned effects. Numerous authors closely associate them or even presume that conditioning is the basic constituent of placebo effects (Ader 1985, Peck & Coleman 1991, Voudoris, Peck & Coleman 1990, Wall 1993, Wickramasekera 1985). However, a differentiation is necessary. Conditioned effects need *specific* presuppositions: first a specific unconditioned stimulus and second a specific setting, which is a very close temporal pairing of the unconditioned and the conditioned stimulus. In many instances, conditioning even seems to work only when it superimposes biological rhythms. These specific presuppositions are usually not present in clinical placebo situations.

Since Pavlov, many experiments on drug-conditioned responses in animals have been carried out. But from these experiments one cannot conclude that *healing* or a real *therapeutic* drug effect also can be provoked as a conditioned reflex. Surely, in cancer patients nausea and vomiting can be conditioned by repeated chemotherapy. But this does not mean that tumour remissions can be conditioned as well. Unfortunately, it is just the other way round: whereas conditioned vomiting often increases during chemotherapy cycles, there is generally a decrease in the therapeutic sensitivity of the tumour.

In fact, clinical experience contradicts the assumption that healing can be conditioned. Episodes of chronic disease are usually more difficult to treat than the acute or first manifestation of an illness, even if this first manifestation has been treated successfully. (Classical conditioning paradigm would predict just the opposite.) Moreover, there are many severe symptoms that are treated effectively by regular and repeated drug administration. These therapeutic settings are similar to conditional settings, and therefore should be adequate for the conditioning of therapeutic effects. Yet when interrupting such regular therapies a rapid deterioration of patients is observed in practice.

Conditioning nevertheless can play a major part in placebo administration, although in an entirely different respect, concerning obliging reports and experimental subordination (Kienle & Kiene 1996). The replies and reports from patients might be susceptible to conditioning, just as it is possible to condition obedience, behaviour and reflexes.

In an example of a crossover placebo-controlled study on hypertension (Suchman & Ader 1992), a conditioned reduction of blood pressure was shown; however, it was short term (a few days). Notably, when placebos were given as first treatment within this crossover design, no antihypertensive effect occurred, although 83% of the patients had previously been treated with antihypertensive remedies. Thus, in this trial (presented as a demonstration of placebo effects) only a short-term conditioned effect occurred, owing to the specific conditioning setting, while there was *no* placebo effect. These findings concur with several trials on placebo in hypertension (Iacono et al 1992, Mancia et al 1995, Report of working party on mild to moderate hypertension

1977, Weber, Neutel & Smith 1995); these did not show any placebo effect either.

Neurotic or psychotic misjudgement

The reliability of a patient's report is often particularly difficult to assess in neurotic or psychotic disturbances (Kienle 1995). Here the placebo literature offers fascinating stories (Schindel 1967). However, one should not forget that a common feature in psychosis or neurosis is disturbed interpretation of reality. Therefore one clearly has to differentiate between a psychotic or neurotic misjudgement on the one hand and a correct observation of a therapeutic effect on the other hand. (This differentiation is difficult, but not impossible; in fact, it is the psychiatrist's daily work.) Neurotic or psychotic misjudgements can hardly give any valid evidence for the existence of placebo effects.

The placebo is not a placebo

How do we know that 'placebos' contain only substances that are inert for the condition in question? How do we rule out the situation where the 'placebo effect' may have been caused by components of the 'placebo' possessing a specific efficacy on the disease that is treated? This question was recently discussed in Nature (Golomb 1995): 'Although the nonspecific effects of placebos are widely studied, the possibility that the chemicals used as placebos may have specific effects has received virtually no attention. ... Astonishingly, no systematic efforts are made to ensure the inertness of placebos. ... The foundation of evidence-based medicine is undermined by the absence of evidence that placebos are inert. It is paradoxical that there is no standard of evidence to support the standard of evidence.'

It is not a rare situation that a 'placebo' treatment possibly contains components that are specifically effective for the condition in question. For example, recently a study reported in the British Medical Journal (Ernst & Resch 1995) tried to determine placebo effects on the basis of clinical trials comparing placebo treated and non-treated patients. Out of 318 trials four were found that showed superior outcomes in the placebo groups. The best trials were two five-armed randomized trials on ultrasound treatment of postoperative swelling after extraction of a wisdom tooth (Hashish, Harvey & Harris 1986, Ho et al 1988). As the placebo group, treated with a turned-off ultrasound apparatus, showed better results than the untreated group the results were categorized as 'true' and 'substantial' placebo effect (Ernst & Resch 1995). However, in the placebo group a coupling cream was also applied, whose cooling effect—due to humidity and increased thermal conductivity—possibly reduced the postoperative swelling. Local cooling must surely be considered to have a specific effect on postoperative swelling. Therefore the 'placebo effect' is questionable, irrespective of the five-arm randomized design.

Another example is an often-quoted placebo effect in surgery, dating back to the 1950s, when the ligation of the internal mammary artery was performed as treatment for angina pectoris. Adams (1958) and Dimond, Kittke & Crockett (1958, 1960) demonstrated that the mere local preparation of the artery without ligation did lead to subjective improvement as well. Consequently, Dimond talked about the 'strong psychotherapy of surgery'. This example is often quoted still today (Johnson 1994, Turner et al 1994) but again the inertness of the placebo treatment is questionable. The operation was started with a local parasternal anaesthesia, and exactly this parasternal injection of a local anaesthetic is the main treatment of all heart diseases in neural therapy (Dosch 1989). According to neural therapy a specific cardiac treatment had been carried out. Thus again, the 'placebo effect' is questionable.

Uncritical reporting of anecdotes

To explain the placebo effect, Beecher (1984) illustrated non-specific or psychological powers by the following story. A middle-aged woman was operated on because of cancer, but the cancer turned out to be inoperable. When the woman recovered from narcosis, one of her relatives told her the truth about her illness. Within the next hour the woman got a cardiovascular shock, and after a few hours she died.

This story, however, is neither a demonstration of any placebo effectiveness, nor is it a demonstration of any unspecific, psychological power. Of course, every rational doctor first would have to rule out the most likely cause, which is a postoperative complication like bleeding or pulmonary embolism. These are frequent complications of operations, particularly in cancer patients, often with fatal outcome.

Misquotations

Wrong quotations are common in the placebo literature. Beecher himself gave essentially incorrect quotations about 10 of his 15 famous trials (Kienle 1995). For instance, he claimed an antitussive placebo effect in 36% of 22 patients, and in 43% of another 22 patients in one of these trials. However, in the original publication (Gravenstein, Devloo & Beecher 1954) no significant change was reported after any of the placebo administrations. There even was no placebo group of 22 patients, and there were no reports about any 43% or 36% of patients. The percentages reported in the original trial referred rather to the amount of a gas volume inhaled by the patients. These completely wrong quotations of Beecher are a surprise, particularly as he himself was one of the authors of the original publication. In other instances, Beecher exaggerated the number of patients treated, or he would state percentages of patients being relieved under placebo. However, in the original publications the percentage numbers did not refer to patients at all but to days of treatment, to numbers of pills given, or to numbers of coughs (Kienle 1995).

A multitude of misquotations can also be found in other placebo literature (Kienle 1995). For example, there is a claim of a positive placebo effect in pain in 67% of patients mentioned in an article by Netter, Classen & Feingold (1986). Netter referred to Janke (1967), Janke referred to Haas, Fink & Härtefelder (1959), who referred to a letter written to the Journal of the American Medical Association (Foreign letters 1957). This letter again referred to an anonymous editorial, which supposedly mentioned a study from another scientist, Kjaer-Larsen, and this Kjaer-Larsen had supposedly reported a 67% quote of patients getting relief under an inert tablet. Within this whole series of quotations no identification of the original trial can be found; one is reminded of a rumour.

Side-effects, toxic reactions

It is claimed that placebos have not only therapeutic effects but side-effects as well, and that they can produce toxic reactions. The reports about side-effects and toxic effects of placebos can be divided into three classes (Kienle 1995).

1. The reports of toxic placebo effects are often based on misquotation. An example is the claim (Joyce 1989, Wolf & Pinsky 1954) of an impressive finding that 61% of the placebo patients in a streptomycin trial showed the specific toxic effects of streptomycin, including high-tone and low-tone hearing loss, eosinophilia and impairment of urea clearance. This remarkable placebo toxicity has been passed on in the medical literature. However, going back to the original publication (Veterans Administration 1948) one finds that *none* of the patients in the streptomycin trial ever received a placebo.

2. Reidenberg & Lowenthal (1968) and Green (1964) showed that many symptoms in many people occur spontaneously, being 'everyday symptoms'. Usually these everyday symptoms remain unnoticed. In the situation of a clinical trial, however, they are documented; this accounts for the placebo group; and thus they are misinterpreted as placebo side-effects. Reidenberg & Lowenthal (1968) asked several hundred healthy young persons who were not taking any medications whether during the last 3 days they had experienced one or more symptoms out of a list of 25. Only 19% of these healthy young people were without symptoms. 30% of them even reported six or more symptoms (see Table 4.2). Similarly, Green (1964)

Table 4.2 Spontaneous occurrence of symptoms in healthy people: percentage of healthy subjects reporting each symptom (Reidenberg & Lowenthal 1968)

Symptom	Group I	Group II
Skin rash	8	3
Urticaria	5	3
Bad dreams	8	3
Excessive sleepiness	23	23
Fatigue	41	37
Inability to concentrate	25	27
Irritability	20	17
Insomnia	7	10
Loss of appetite	3	6
Dry mouth	5	3
Nausea	3	2
Vomiting	0	0
Diarrhoea	5	2
Constipation	4	3
Palpitations	3	3
Giddiness or weakness	2	3
Faintness or dizziness on first standing up	5	5
Headaches	15	13
Fever	3	1
Pain in joints	9	5
Pain in muscles	10	11
Nasal congestion	31	13
Bleeding or bruising	3	3
Bleeding from gums after brushing teeth	21	20
Excessive bleeding from gums after brushing teeth	1	1

screened 4408 subjects (penitentiary inmates, professional personnel, aged inmates in a home, medical patients) for symptoms typical of so-called 'side-effects' before and after a placebo administration. Pretreatment 'side-effects' were frequent in all groups. After placebos were administered the incidence of the so-called 'side-effects' increased slightly amongst healthy people, while it decreased in the group of aged inmates and remained similar in the patients. Altogether, the data indicated spontaneous fluctuation of pre-existing symptoms, but no placebo effects. Green (1964) concluded: 'These findings suggested that the effects found had been influenced by what the investigator was looking for, with the possibility that pre-existing conditions, which otherwise could have gone unnoticed, were being uncovered and regarded as side effects.'

Most of the reported placebo side-effects have the same frequency and the same characteristics as spontaneous everyday symptoms. Therefore it is very probable that the so-called placebo side-effects are not effects of placebo administration, but spontaneously varying everyday symptoms.

3. Sometimes symptoms are called side-effects of placebos when diseases were treated with placebos but symptoms did not get any better.

For example, drowsiness, diarrhoea, nausea and vomiting occurring in patients with irritable colon were classified as 'side-effects' of placebo administration, without considering that these might be symptoms of irritable colon itself that simply did not improve through placebo treatment (Kasich, Fein & Miller 1959).

CONCLUSION

It is generally assumed that the administration of an inert pill can have therapeutic effects in one-third or more of all patients in a variety of diseases. The healing power of an inert tablet—'the lie that heals' (Brody 1982), or 'the power of a sugar pill' (Evans 1974)—is considered a well-proven scientific fact. However, contrary to the widely held belief that placebo effects in pharmacotherapy have been universally and scientifically demonstrated, no *therapeutic placebo effect* has been demonstrated credibly in any of the studies analysed (Kienle 1995, Kienle & Kiene 1996, 1997). The same accounts for time–effect curves of placebo administration, accumulation and carry-over effects, and differentiated actions depending on colour, size or packaging (Kienle & Kiene 1996). Only in bronchial asthma have suggestion effects, combined with placebo administration, been documented under experimental conditions (Kienle & Kiene 1996), but whether placebo treatment of asthmatic symptoms is feasible under clinical conditions remains an open question.

Possibly placebo effects in experimental pain have been demonstrated; a trial by Benedetti (1996) recently showed short-term (1-hour) effects within a sophisticated study design. Still, many questions remain concerning this trial. For example, the strongest analgesic 'effect' under placebo administration was observed when placebo had been applied *unnoticed*.

After carrying out our analysis, we ourselves have come to the conclusion that the widespread data in the literature on the magnitude and frequency of the placebo effect are largely exaggerated, if not altogether false. They are the expression of an irrational 'placebo euphoria' already emphasized by Hollister (1960) in his essay 'Placebology: sense and nonsense'. He writes that although in general we have a very critical attitude to reports of the effects of a drug, reports of seeming placebo effects always arouse great enthusiasm and uncritical acceptance. In our opinion, one must ask whether the existence of the so-called placebo effect—'the lie that heals', therapy through deceit—is largely, if not entirely, an illusion.

The many false assessments made in this field are due not only to documentary and methodological negligence, but also to a lack of conceptual differentiation. The concept of the placebo, which gained most of its great medicohistorical acceptance in the 1940s and 1950s in the field of pharmacotherapy (Beecher 1955, Conferences on therapy 1946, Pepper 1945), primarily referred to the *imitation of a therapy*. However, after quantifying the presumed power of the inert tablet the concept was immediately extended to embrace psychotherapy, creative therapy, and all kinds of psychological influences on physical events within the concept of the placebo. If our analyses erase doubts about the existence of the placebo effect in its narrow sense (i.e. true *therapeutic* effects achieved by mere *imitation* of a therapy), it does not rule out the possibility that the patient's self-healing powers may be influenced by a wide variety of non-pharmacological approaches. In our opinion, one should be particularly cautious about dismissing therapeutic procedures used in other cultures. To us, it seems inappropriate to call such therapeutic approaches simply 'placebos'. Such a label may all too easily mask our own ignorance and lack of understanding when research and attempts at understanding would be more appropriate. Borkovec (1985) emphasized this as much as 10 years ago: 'In some circumstances and in the absence of existing theories, we certainly may choose to look up from our bewildered mental state and say the effect was due to "placebo". But we probably would benefit from avoiding a feeling of satisfaction from so doing. Our real task is to continue exploring effects that we do not understand.'

REFERENCES

Adams R 1958 Internal-mammary-artery ligation for coronary insufficiency: an evaluation. New England Journal of Medicine 258:113–115
Ader R 1985 Conditioned immunopharmacological effects in animals: implications for a conditioning model of pharmacotherapy. In: White L, Tursky B, Schwartz G E (eds) Placebo—theory, research, and mechanisms. Guilford, New York, 306–323
Albert H 1991 Traktat über die kritische Vernunft. Mohr, Tübingen
Barber T X 1963 The effects of 'hypnosis' on pain. Psychosomatic Medicine 25:303–333
Beecher H K 1955 The powerful placebo. Journal of the American Medical Association 159:1602–1606
Beecher H K 1984 Die Placebowirkung als unspezifischer Wirkungsfaktor im Bereich der Krankheit und der Krankenbehandlung. In: Gross F, Beecher H K (eds) Placebo—das universelle Medikament? Eggebrecht-Presse, Mainz
Beecher H K, Deffer P A, Fink F E, Sullivan D B 1951 Field use of methadone and levo-isomethadone in a combat zone. US Armed Forces Medical Journal II:1269–1276
Beecher H K, Keats A S, Mosteller F, Lasagna L 1953 The effectiveness of oral analgesics (morphine, codeine, acetylsalicylic acid) and the problem of placebo 'reactors' and 'non-reactors'. Journal of Pharmacology and Experimental Therapeutics 109:393–400
Benedetti F 1996 The opposite effects of the opiate antagonist naloxone and the cholecystokinin antagonist proglumide on placebo analgesia. Pain 64:535–543
Blomberg L H 1957 Treatment of disseminated sclerosis with active and inactive drugs. Lancet i:431–432
Bodem S H 1994 Bedeutung der Placebowirkung in der praktischen Arzneitherapie. Pharmacologische Zeitung 139:9–19
Borkovec T D 1985 Defining the unknown. In: White L, Tursky B, Schwartz G E (eds) Placebo—theory, research, and mechanisms. Guilford, New York, pp 59–64
Brody H 1982 The lie that heals: the ethics of giving placebos. Annals of Internal Medicine 97:112–118
Byrd R C 1988 Positive therapeutic effects of intercessory prayer in a coronary care unit population. Southern Medical Journal 81:826–829

Clark W C 1969 Sensory-decision theory analysis of the effect on the criterion for pain and thermal sensitivity. Journal of Abnormal Psychology 74:363–371

Coe W S, Best M M, Kinsman J M 1950 Veratrum viride in the treatment of hypertensive vascular disease. Journal of the American Medical Association 143:5–7

Conferences on therapy 1946 The use of placebos in therapy. New York State Journal of Medicine August:1718–1727

Deyo R A 1993 Practice variations, treatment fads, rising disability. Spine 18:2153–2216

Diehl H S 1993 Medical treatment of the common cold. Journal of the American Medical Association 101:2042–2049

Dimond E G, Kittle C F, Crockett J E 1958 Evaluation of internal mammary artery ligation and sham procedure in angina pectoris. Circulation 18:712–713

Dimond E G, Kittle C F, Crockett J E 1960 Comparison of internal mammary artery ligation and sham operation for angina pectoris. American Journal of Cardiology 5:483–486

Dosch P 1989 Lehrbuch der Neuraltherapie nach Huneke. Karl F. Haug Verlag, Heidelberg

Dossey L, Schellhorn W 1995 Heilende Worte (trans.) Verlag Bruno Martin, Sudergellersen

Dyken M, White P T 1956 Evaluation of cortisone in the treatment of cerebral infarction. Journal of the American Medical Association 162:1531–1534

Ernst E, Resch K L 1995 Concept of true and perceived placebo effects. British Medical Journal 311:551–553

Evans F J 1974 The power of a sugar pill. Psychology Today April:55–59

Evans W, Hoyle C 1933 The comparative value of drugs used in the continuous treatment of angina pectoris. Quarterly Journal of Medicine 7:311–338

Fordyce W E, Lansky D, Calsyn D A, Shelton J L, Stolov W C, Rock D L 1984 Pain measurement and pain behavior. Pain 18:53–69

Foreign letters 1957 Journal of the American Medical Association 163:674

Gay L N, Carliner P E 1949 The prevention and treatment of motion sickness. Bulletin of the Johns Hopkins Hospital 84:470–487

Golomb B A 1995 Paradox of the placebo effect. Nature 375:530

Gøtzsche P C 1994 Is there logic in the placebo? Lancet 344:925–926

Gravenstein J S, Devloo R A, Beecher H K 1954 Effect of antitussive agents on experimental and pathological cough in man. Journal of Applied Physiology 7:119–139

Green D M 1964 Pre-existing conditions, placebo reactions, and 'side effects'. Annals of Internal Medicine 60:255–265

Greiner T, Gold H, Cattell M et al 1950 A method for the evaluation of the effects of drugs on cardiac pain in patients with angina of effort. A study of khellin (visammin). American Journal of Medicine 9:143–155

Haas H, Fink H, Härtefelder G 1959 Das Placeboproblem. In: Jucker E (ed) Fortschritte der Arzneimittelforschung. Birkhäuser, Basel, pp 279–454

Hashish I, Harvey W, Harris M 1986 Anti-inflammatory effects of ultrasound therapy: evidence for a major placebo effect. British Journal of Rheumatology 25:77–81

Hillis B R 1952 The assessment of cough-suppressing drugs. Lancet June 21:1230–1235

Ho K H, Hashish I, Salmon P, Freeman R, Harvey W 1988 Reduction of post-operative swelling by a placebo effect. Journal of Psychosomatic Research 32:197–205

Hollister L 1960. Placebology: sense and nonsense. Current Therapy Research 2:477–483

Hornung J 1994 Was ist ein Placebo? Die Bedeutung einer korrekten Definition für die klinische Forschung. Fortschritte der Komplementärmedizin 1:160–165

Iacono P, Drici M D, De Lunardo C, Salimbeni B, Lapalus P 1992 Placebo effect in cardiovascular clinical pharmacology. International Journal of Clinical Pharmacology Research XII:53–56

Janke W 1967 Experimentelle Untersuchungen zur psychischen Wirkung von Placebos bei gesunden Probanden. Mathematisch-Naturwissenschaftliche Fakultät der Universität Gießen

Jellinek E M 1946 Clinical tests on comparative effectiveness of analgesic drugs. Biometrics 2:87–91

Johnson A G 1994 Surgery as a placebo. Lancet 344:1140–1142

Joyce C R B 1989 Non-specific aspects of treatment from the point of view of a clinical pharmacologist. In: Shepherd M, Sartorius N (eds) Non-specific aspects of treatment. Huber, Bern, pp 57–94

Kasich A M, Fein H D, Miller J W 1959 Comparative effect of phenaglycodol, meprobamate, and a placebo on the irritable colon. American Journal of Digestive Diseases 4:229–234

Keats A S, Beecher H K 1950 Pain relief with hypnotic doses of barbiturates and a hypothesis. Journal of Pharmacology and Experimental Therapeutics 100:1–13

Keats A S, D'Alessandro G L, Beecher H K 1951 A controlled study of pain relief by intravenous procaine. Journal of the American Medical Association 147:1761–1763

Kiene H 1993 Kritik der klinischen Doppelblindstudie. München: MMV Medizin Verlag

Kiene H 1996 A critique of the double-blind clinical trial. Alternative Therapies in Health and Medicine 2:59–64, 74–80

Kienle G S 1995 Der sogenannte Placeboeffekt; Illusion, Fakten, Realität. Schattauer Verlag GmbH, Stuttgart

Kienle G S, Kiene H 1996 Placebo effect and placebo concept: a critical methodological and conceptual analysis of reports on the magnitude of the placebo effect. Alternative Therapies in Health and Medicine 2:39–54

Kienle G S, Kiene H 1997 The powerful placebo effect. Fact or fiction? Journal of Clinical Epidemiology 50:1311–1318

Lasagna L, Mosteller F, Felsinger J M, Beecher H K 1954 A study of the placebo response. American Journal of Medicine 16:770–779

Lasagna L, Felsinger J M, Beecher H K 1955 Drug-induced mood changes in man. 1. Observations on healthy subjects, chronically ill patients, and 'postaddicts'. Journal of the American Medical Association 157:1006–1020

LeRoy G V 1941 The effectiveness of the xanthine drugs in the treatment of angina pectoris. Journal of the American Medical Association 116:921–925

Liberman R 1962 An analysis of the placebo phenomenon. Journal of Chronic Disease 15:761–783

Lichstein J, DeCosta Mayer J, Hauch E W 1955 Efficacy of methantheline (banthine) bromide in therapy of the unstable colon. Journal of the American Medical Association June 25:634–637

Long D M, Uematsu S, Kouba R B 1989 Placebo responses to medical device therapy for pain. Stereotactic and Functional Neurosurgery 53:149–156

McDonald C, Mazzuca S, McCabe G 1983 How much of the placebo 'effect' is really statistical regression? Statistical Medicine 2:417–427

Mancia G, Omboni S, Parati G, Ravogli A, Villani A, Zanchetti A 1995 Lack of placebo effect on ambulatory blood pressure. American Journal of Health 8:311–315

Meyer U A, Kindli R 1989 Plazebos und Nozebos. Therapeutische Umschau 46:544–554

Moerman D E 1983 General medical effectiveness and human biology: placebos effects in the treatment of ulcer disease. Medical Anthropology Quarterly 14:13–16

Netter P, Classen W, Feingold E 1986 Das Placeboproblem. In: Dölle W, Müller-Oerlinghausen B, Schwabe U (eds) Grundlagen der Arzneimitteltherapie—Entwicklung, Beurteilung und Anwendung von Arzneimitteln. Wissenschaftsverlag, Mannheim, pp 355–366

Peck C, Coleman G 1991 Implications of placebo theory for clinical research and practice in pain management. Theoretical Medicine 12:247–270

Pepper O H P 1945 A note on placebo. Annals of the Journal of Pharmacy 117:409–412

Reidenberg M M, Lowenthal D T 1968 Adverse nondrug reactions. New England Journal of Medicine 279:678–679

Report of research council working party on mild to moderate hypertension 1977 Randomized controlled trial of treatment for mild hypertension: design and pilot trial. British Medical Journal 1:1437–1440

Roberts A H 1995 The powerful placebo revisited: the magnitude of nonspecific effects. Mind/Body Medicine March: 1–1

Roberts A H, Kewman D G, Mercier L, Hovell M 1993 The power of nonspecific effects in healing: implications for psychosocial and biological treatments. Clinical Psychology Review 13:375–391

Sackett D L 1995 Randomized trials in individual patients. In: Antes G, Edler L, Holle R, Köpcke W, Lorenz R, Windeler J (eds) Biometrie und unkonventionelle Medizin. Landwirtschaftsverlag GmbH, Münster-Hiltrup, pp 19–33

Schindel L 1967 Placebo und Placebo-Effekte in Klinik und Forschung. Arzneimittelforschung 17:892–918

Suchman A L, Ader R 1992 Classic conditioning and placebo effects in crossover studies. Clinical Pharmacological Therapy 52:372–337

Tedeschi J T, Schlenker B R, Bonoma T V 1971 Cognitive dissonance: private ratiocination or public spectacle? American Psychologist 26:685–695

Travell J, Rinzler S H, Bakst H, Benjamin Z H, Bobb A 1949 A comparison of effects of alpha-tocopherol and a matching placebo on chest pain in patients with heart disease. Annals of the New York Academy of Sciences 52:345–353

Turner J A, Deyo R A, Loeser J D, Von Korff M, Fordyce W E 1994 The importance of placebo effects in pain treatment and research. Journal of the American Medical Association 271:1609–1614

Veterans Administration 1948 Minutes of the Fifth Streptomycin Conference. Knickerbocker Hotel, Chicago, IL

Voudouris N J, Peck C L, Coleman G 1990 The role of conditioning and verbal expectancy in the placebo response. Pain 43:121–128

Wall P D 1993 Pain and the placebo response. Ciba Foundation Symposium 174:187–211

Weber M A, Neutel J M, Smith D H G 1995 Controlling blood pressure throughout the day: issues in testing a new anti-hypertensive agent. Journal of Human Hypertension 9 (suppl 5):29–35

Whitney C W, Von Korff M 1992 Regression to the mean in treated versus untreated chronic pain. Pain 50:281–285

Wickramasekera I 1985 A conditioned response model of the placebo effect: predictions from the model. In: White L, Tursky B, Schwartz G E (eds) Placebo—theory, research, and mechanisms, Guilford, New York, pp 255–287

Wolf S, Pinsky R H 1954 Effects of placebo administration and the occurrence of toxic reactions. Journal of the American Medical Association 155:339–341

4

Behavioural conditioning of the immune system

Angela Clow

Editor's note

It was an experimental study of conditioning effects that launched the whole field of psychoneuroimmunology. When I first learned in the early eighties that Robert Ader had (inadvertently) conditioned a down-regulation of his laboratory rats' immune system, it was like hearing the missing link had been discovered. Dr Clow deftly overviews the short history of PNI, leading us into a fascinating territory of pathways that translate psychological experiences into physiological and pathophysiological change. This chapter begins to put pieces of the jigsaw together: mind, brain, stress, self-healing and immunity. She demonstrates just how far we have come from the idea that non-pharmacological therapeutic effects are simply 'all in the mind'. For there is more to the new psychosomatics than that: if the term formerly implied that the mind can undermine well-being, then here she presents some of the experimental evidence for beneficial psychosomatic processes. Does this mean mainstream medicine could embrace a scientific approach to triggering self-healing? Could they be integrated into conventional treatment—even, as research alluded to here suggests, into high-tech areas such as cancer chemotherapy? This chapter gives grounds for believing that the term 'placebo' response may disguise quite specific effects, and this has important implications for our understanding of complementary and mind–body therapies.

The study of the relationship between the brain and immune system has given rise to the interdisciplinary area of research known as psychoneuroimmunology, or PNI. As the name suggests this area explores how psychological affect (emotion) can mediatc changes in immune function, and hence susceptibility to certain illness, via brain and nervous system mechanisms. The placebo effect involves changes in physical signs and symptoms (often involving aspects of the immune system) in relation to the belief of the patient. In this respect the placebo effect can be viewed as a physical response to a change in psychological affect and provides a demonstration of the power of PNI in everyday life. The impact of stress and depression on aspects of immunity and susceptibility to illness is now well established. Any placebo agent or procedure capable of reducing either of these psychological states is thus likely to lessen their impact on the immune system and hence moderate related illness. Indeed it is probable that much of the success of early medical practitioners relied on their ability to relieve anxiety, by careful description of the disease process, rather than on active treatment. In this chapter I explore another important mechanism by which the placebo effect may be mediated—that is, behavioural conditioning of the immune system. First, however, I shall briefly expand on the evidence that the brain is central in the relationship between psychological affect and aspects of immunity.

THE BRAIN HEMISPHERES AND IMMUNITY

The case is made, elsewhere in this book (Ch. 14), that the brain mediates the relationship between emotion (stress and depression) and immunity. In this chapter I concentrate on the postulated differential role for each side of the brain in regulation of immune function. There is a widely held belief that, at the most basic level, motivation and emotion can be categorized as either 'positive' or 'negative' and that the left and the right brain can be associated with these emotions and resultant behaviours (i.e. 'approach' and 'withdrawal' respectively). It follows therefore, given what we know about the relationship between emotion and the immune system, that activation of each hemisphere (different emotions) will have differential effects on the immune system. There is much evidence to suggest that this is the case and that in 'normally' lateralized individuals the left hemisphere may be preferentially associated with activation of cell-mediated immunity whereas the right hemispheres may be preferentially associated with humoral immunity.

The role of the hemispheres in emotion

Some of the first evidence for a differential role for the hemispheres in emotion was derived from clinical observation. Patients who had suffered unilateral left-hemisphere brain damage/loss of function (right hemisphere intact) tended to experience more feelings of despair, hopelessness or anger compared with patients who had similar but right-hemisphere damage. In contrast, right-hemisphere damage (with the left hemisphere intact) was observed to be associated with 'indifference—euphoric reaction' in which (perhaps surprisingly) minimization of symptoms, emotional placidity and elation were common (Gainotti 1969). Consistent with these findings were the results from non-traumatized individuals subjected to the Wada test (where one hemisphere is anaesthetized). Anaesthetization of the left hemisphere (so only the right hemisphere is active) tended to cause dysphoric reactions (e.g. crying), whereas the same procedure to the right (so only the left hemisphere is active) was associated with euphoria and feelings of well-being (e.g. laughing) (Rossi & Rosadini 1967, Terzian 1964).

These observations were systematically explored in the laboratory by electrophysiologists who could measure activity in the brain by using recording electrodes placed on the skull. This work showed that the left and right hemispheres were indeed differentially active during positive and negative emotion. The left frontal region was activated during positive, approach-related emotion whereas the right frontal cortex was more activated during negative, withdrawal-related emotion (Davidson & Sutton 1995).

Individual differences were observed in the asymmetrical activity of the frontal cerebral cortex during periods of no emotional experience and it was proposed that we can all be classified according to whether we are predominately 'right'- or 'left'-brain-dominant individuals. 'Left-brain-active' individuals were characterized by more intense positive emotion to emotionally positive stimuli whereas 'right-brain-active' subjects tended to react with more intense negative emotion to emotionally negative stimuli (Wheeler, Davidson & Tomarken 1993). In addition, subjects with greater basal left-brain activation tended to be more positive generally and minimize negative affect in their daily lives (in a similar way to the right-brain-damaged patients described above) (Tomarken & Davidson 1994, Tomarken et al 1992). Importantly, those subjects who showed predominately higher resting left-frontal-cortex activation had significantly higher levels of NK-cell activity compared with predominately right-hemisphere-active individuals. On the other hand, predominately right-active subjects had higher levels of the antibody immunoglobulin M (Kang et al 1991). (See Ch. 14 for a detailed description of immune cells.) These data support the left: cell-mediated/right: humoral-mediated hypothesis outlined above.

Cerebral lateralization and immune function

Lymphocyte function

Recently it has been shown that lymphocyte function is related to cerebral lateralization. The language-dominant hemisphere of patients undergoing surgery for epilepsy was determined and immune status measured before and after surgery. There was a reduction in T-cell indices (peripheral circulating total T cells including both CD4+ and CD8+ T cells) only in those patients who received surgery on the language-dominant hemisphere. There was an increase in these indices following surgery in the non-language-dominant hemisphere (Meador et al 1999). This study provides additional evidence to support the view that the left hemisphere may mediate up-regulation of cell-mediated immunity. If the left hemisphere is damaged then that regulation is impaired and T-cell indices are reduced. If the right hemisphere is damaged the left hemisphere can prevail over the restraining influence of the right, and T-cell indices rise. Subjects with reduced left-hemisphere domination tend to lean toward humoral-mediated immunity and immunoglobulin E (IgE) hypersensitivity atopic responses.

Disease progression

The significance of these differences in immune function, mediated by cerebral lateralization, to health has been investigated in terms of disease progression. Asymptomatic HIV-positive men have been followed up for 30 months. It is known that AIDS progression is associated with a shift from cell-mediated to humoral immunity (Clerici & Shearer 1994). It was found that those individuals with greater left cerebral dominance maintained proportionally greater cell-mediated immunity for longer and this was associated with a slower disease progression and better mood (Gruzelier et al 1996). It seems therefore that lateralized control of immune function is not a redundant irrelevancy but may be fundamental to disease susceptibility.

Secretory immunoglobulin activity

It is known that pleasant and unpleasant odours can differentially activate areas of the left and right cerebral cortex respectively (work demonstrated by recording brain activity through the skull (Martin 1998). This knowledge was utilized to explore the effect of odours on the secretion of secretory immunoglobulin A (sIgA). sIgA is an antibody that is secreted across all of the body's mucosal surfaces and provides a barrier to invasion by pathogen. Levels of sIgA have been shown to be very sensitive to psychological affect as well as affecting susceptibility to infection. In this particular experiment subjects were blindfolded and unaware of what odour they were about to be exposed to. Presentation of the pleasant smell of chocolate (known to activate the left hemisphere) caused increased sIgA secretion whereas presentation of the unpleasant smell of rotten meat (right-hemisphere activation) caused the opposite effect (Clow et al in preparation).

The effect was immediate (during presentation of the odour) and transient (gone 10 minutes later). So this experiment suggested that the left-hemisphere activation was associated with increased transport of the antibody sIgA across the mucosal surfaces.

THE ROLE OF THE AUTONOMIC NERVOUS SYSTEM

It is probable that any association between the brain, emotion and the immune system is mediated via the autonomic nervous system (ANS). The sympathetic branch of the ANS, in particular, is known to have important influences on lymphoid tissue and the lymphocytes it produces. Predictably, perhaps, asymmetrical hemispheric regulation of the ANS has been demonstrated. Substantial evidence to this effect has been derived from direct brain stimulation during neurosurgery. Stimulation of the insula cortex in the left hemisphere resulted in bradycardia (slowing of the heartbeat) whereas right insular stimulation caused tachycardia (increased heartbeat) (Oppenheimer et al 1992). Consistent with this finding, right-hemisphere pathology (stroke), resulting in reduced function, has been associated with reduced sympathetic activation (Sander & Klingelhofer 1995). Similarly experimental stroke in cats and rats have provided evidence of right-sided dominance for sympathetic effects (Cechetto 1993). Thus it is probable that asymmetrical cortical regulation of immune function may be mediated via an asymmetric ANS. Indeed the evidence suggests that sympathetic activation (dominant from the right hemisphere) will shift the balance of the immune system in favour of humoral immunity, which is consistent with the hypothesis presented here.

NEUROTRANSMITTER EFFECTS

In addition, asymmetrical distribution of the monoamine neurotransmitters in the two hemispheres has been demonstrated. This group of neurotransmitters includes dopamine, noradrenaline and serotonin, which provide the pivotal link between mood and the immune system. Dopamine is the brain's main 'reward substance'. Addictive drugs like cocaine dramatically increase levels of dopamine in the brain. The other two monoamines (noradrenaline and serotonin) have been intimately linked to mood: too-high levels of these are associated with anxiety whereas reduced levels are linked with depression (the antidepressant drug Prozac works to boost brain serotonin levels). The point is that these neurotransmitters are key chemicals in mood and motivation. Bearing in mind what is known about the asymmetrical brain regulation of these psychological domains it is perhaps predictable that they too are asymmetrically distributed: higher concentrations of dopamine are found in the left hemisphere (approach motivation, pleasure) and higher concentrations of the other two in the right (withdrawal motivation, anxiety) (Barnoud, Le Moal & Neveu 1990).

THE HPA AXIS

Apart from the ANS the other major system capable of affecting the immune system is the hypothalamic–pituitary–adrenal (HPA) axis. The observed increase in circulating levels of the product of HPA activation— that is, cortisol (in humans)—following mood manipulation (usually unpleasant) provides evidence for this. The link here is that activity of the HPA axis is largely dependent upon relative levels of the monoamine neurotransmitters described above. Critically, central noradrenaline and serotonin can initiate the HPA cascade to cause release of cortisol. As the right hemisphere is especially rich in these neurotransmitters it can be hypothesized that this hemisphere dominates in regulation of the HPA axis. High levels of circulating cortisol have an impact on the balance of the immune system. In short, cortisol promotes a shift to humoral immunity, away from cell-mediated immunity. Thus differential activation of the HPA axis by the two hemispheres provides another mechanism for the immunomodulatory effects of cerebral lateralization.

There is some direct evidence that the HPA axis is asymmetrically regu- lated in the direction suggested above. However, much less work has been carried out in this area, compared with that on asymmetrical regulation of the immune system itself. This is probably because explanatory mecha- nisms are usually explored after establishment of the initial phenomenon. However, the available evidence does point to right-hemisphere domina- tion for glucocorticoid (e.g. cortisol) production. Rodent studies have demonstrated that removal of parts of the right cerebral cortex leads to down-regulation of both basal and stress-induced glucocorticoid levels whereas removal of the identical area of the left hemisphere has no effect (Sullivan & Gratton 1999). In humans it has been shown that presentation of an aversive video (electroconvulsive treatment of a patient) to either the right or left visual field produced greater cortisol responses following right hemifield presentation (Wittling & Pfluger 1990). This result could not be attributed to the video simply eliciting a greater emotional response following right-side presentation. Thus these data are consistent with right-side dominance for activation of the HPA axis.

BEHAVIOURAL CONDITIONING AND PLACEBO EFFECTS

The evidence above demonstrates that the brain can influence immune processes in a lateralized, asymmetrical way that is related to motivation and mood is a powerful tenet of PNI. The link between emotion and immu- nity is not assumed or spurious, but real and significant to all our lives. All emotion is experienced in and mediated by parts of the brain and the brain has links with the immune system via the autonomic nervous system and HPA axis. Differential activation of emotions (and hence the brain) can modulate the balance of the immune system between cell-mediated and humoral immunity and consequently determine susceptibility to disease types. It is not surprising therefore that the immune system is susceptible to the power of 'belief' and that this influence may play an important role in the placebo effect.

Experimental studies on pavlovian conditioning

The discovery that the immune system could be behaviourally conditioned provided yet further evidence of the link between brain and immunity and is another cornerstone of modern PNI. However the clinical significance of classical pavlovian conditioning on the immune system, including its contribution to the placebo effect, is only now beginning to be fully appreciated. The fact that the immune system can be conditioned (i.e. learn to respond to a neutral stimulus that had been previously paired with a stimulus with direct effects on some aspect of immunity) was first discovered in the mid 1970s. The early work explored this phenomenon using rigorously controlled experiments in animals, mainly rodents. More recently it has been demonstrated that humans respond in the same way. Indeed, anecdotal clinical observation of such conditioning first appeared in the literature over 100 years ago: a paper rose was observed to induce an allergic reaction in a susceptible individual (Mackenzie 1896). Similarly, it has been reported that the picture of a hay field was sufficient to elicit a hay fever attack in very sensitive subjects (Hill 1930). Experimental exposure to symbolic, non-allergenic environmental stimuli previously associated with allergenic stimuli was also able to induce asthmatic symptoms in both animals and some human subjects (Khan 1977, Ottenberg et al 1958). It is now widely accepted that neutral associative processes (agents and procedures) can modify the immune system and that this is under the control of the brain, central nervous and neuroendocrine systems. Furthermore, studies have revealed that such conditioning is both commonplace in the clinical setting and significant in terms of disease progression. Taken together with the evidence that psychological affect and even differential activation of the left and right hemispheres can influence the immune system, these studies were fundamental in the establishment of PNI.

Conditioned taste suppression

Classical pavlovian conditioning theory states that pairing of an active agent (unconditioned stimulus or UCS) with a neutral agent (conditioned stimulus or CS) can result in the neutral agent acquiring the properties of the active agent. Ader & Cohen (1975) were the first to demonstrate that this could happen in the immune system. In fact their original experiment did not set out to investigate this phenomenon. They were primarily interested in conditioned taste aversion. They provided fluid-deprived rats with access to a palatable distinctly flavoured, but harmless, drinking solution (containing saccharin) 30 minutes prior to an injection of toxic agent capable of making the animals feel unwell (owing to temporary gastrointestinal upset). When the rats were re-exposed to the palatable and harmless saccharin solution their consumption was severely reduced. In their experimental paradigm the rats associated a saccharin solution with feeling unwell so they avoided drinking it—this was conditioned taste aversion.

Conditioned immunosuppression

One of the drugs Ader & Cohen used (cyclophosphamide: CY) in the above experiments coincidentally also possessed immunosuppressive properties. The crucial observation was that some animals died and that these were the animals that had consumed the largest volume of saccharin solution during the conditioning trial (all animals received equal amounts of CY). As the saccharin could not have induced the premature death Ader & Cohen hypothesized that the pairing of saccharin with the immunosuppressive agent resulted in conditioning of immunosuppression (as well as taste aversion). Thus, in the conditioned animals the more saccharin consumed the more immunosuppressed they became. Such immunosuppressed animals would be more vulnerable to latent pathogens and hence premature death.

Ader & Cohen went on to explore the phenomenon and test their hypothesis. As is customary in classical-conditioning paradigms, the animals were maintained in a deprived state prior to pairing the unconditioned and conditioned stimuli. Thus following a period of adaptation to a water deprivation (i.e. access to water for only 15 minutes per day) animals were presented with the solution of saccharin and 30 minutes later given an injection of immunosuppressive agent. For up to 6 days after conditioning they were tested for immunosuppression by means of quantifying the antibody response to antigen challenge. The results were as the researchers had predicted. Conditioned animals previously exposed to a single dose of CY paired with the saccharin solution showed a significantly reduced antibody response compared with both saline-treated, non-conditioned animals and conditioned animals (saccharin paired with CY) not subsequently exposed to the saccharin.

Taste aversion alone could not account for the observed effects on the immune system as administration of an aversive but non-immunosuppressive agent (lithium chloride) induced taste aversion without immunosuppression. The results provided clear evidence for the existence of behaviourally conditioned immunosuppression. Many experiments followed. The conclusion was that conditioned immunosuppression was a robust phenomenon that could be demonstrated across a variety of experimental paradigms (see Cohen, Moynihan & Ader 1994). For example, animals conditioned using injection of the immunosuppressive agent cyclosporine A (CsA) as the UCS displayed significant reductions in thymus, spleen and lymphoid organ weights when re-presented with the CS (saccharin solution). This effect could last for up to seven re-presentations following an initial pairing of three consecutive trials (Exton et al 1998a). Conditioned changes in immune function could also be obtained without observable conditioned avoidance responses and were not confined to use of a single unconditioned stimulus. Indeed, it was shown that it was not even necessary to use an immunosuppressive chemical agent to elicit these effects: conditioned suppression of antibody-mediated responses has been obtained using electric shock as the UCS.

Changes in cell-mediated immunity

Conditioned immunosuppression is not restricted to the humoral branch of the immune system; changes in cell-mediated immunity have also been demonstrated. Indeed, conditioning within the immune system may be mediated by a preferential effect on T cells. For example, in rodents, conditioned suppression of lymphoproliferative responses are more robust following administration of T-cell mitogens compared with those for B-cell mitogens (see Ader & Cohen 1993). Stress, in the form of electric footshock (the UCS), paired with either auditory or visual cues (the CS) has been shown to cause a conditioned reduction in activity of natural killer (NK) cells (Perez & Lysle 1997). The effect on T cells in immune system conditioning may be mediated through the cell-mediated cytokine interleukin 2 (IL2). This cytokine is particularly sensitive to conditioning paradigms. Investigators have demonstrated conditioned decreases in IL2 production that could account for suppression of T-cell proliferation. Although replacement of IL2 did not normalize conditioned immunosuppression, IL2 receptors have been shown to be down-regulated, which suggests compromised ability to respond to IL2 may be the key (Exton et al 1998b). Moreover the conditioned reduction in cytokine production (induced using CsA as the US and saccharin solution as the CS) could be completely abrogated by surgical denervation of the spleen (cutting the splenic nerve). Thus it can be concluded that the nervous system, rather than bloodborne products (like glucocorticoids), is primarily instrumental in conditioning this aspect of immune function (Exton et al 1998b). Furthermore, although parallel conditioning of both the HPA axis and aspects of immunity has been demonstrated these two events do not appear to be causally related.

The time course for extinction of the conditioned responses in these two systems is not the same (Buske-Kirschbaum et al 1996).

Antibody production

More recently it has been demonstrated that immuno*suppression* is not uniquely susceptible to conditioning. The *production* of serum antibody to antigen can also be classically conditioned. Animals exposed to a defined antigen (the UCS) in association with a taste-conditioned stimulus (CS) could induce antibody (IgM and IgG) on re-exposure to the CS (Alvarez-Borda et al 1995). Similarly NK-cell numbers and activity have also been shown to be susceptible to *enhancement* by conditioning (Ghanta et al 1996). Even the somewhat impaired immune system of aged animals has been shown to be susceptible to immune conditioning (Spector et al 1994). These interesting findings demonstrate the possibility of conditioning immune responses in young and old alike, offering a valuable tool for attenuating age-related immune deterioration in various species, including humans.

CLINICAL SIGNIFICANCE OF IMMUNE CONDITIONING

The question as to whether such conditioning has any biological or clinical significance still remains to be addressed. Evidence for clinical effects exists in both animals and humans.

Experimental studies in animals

The effect of conditioned immunosuppression on a strain of mice that shows a genetic predisposition to develop systemic lupus-erythematosus-like autoimmune disease has been investigated. Conditioned stimuli were substituted for half of the weekly treatments of active immunosuppressive drugs. Importantly the conditioned response was successful in delaying the onset of the disease, when used in conjunction with normally ineffective doses of drug (Ader & Cohen 1982). Also in lupus-prone mice previously conditioned animals re-exposed to the CS (saccharin) prolonged survival relative to those animals that were not re-exposed to the CS (Ader 1985). Similar beneficial results have been obtained in an animal model of rheumatoid arthritis (Klosterhalfen & Klosterhalfen 1983).

Conditioned immunosuppression has also been shown to be beneficial in retarding rejection of transplant tissues in animals (Gorczynski 1990). Similarly the survival of heart allografts in rats could be prolonged by behaviourally conditioned immunosuppression (Grochowicz et al 1991). On the other hand, as one would predict, animals conditioned to show immunosuppression to a CS showed accelerated mortality when exposed to cancer-provoking agents (Gorczynski, Kennedy & Ciampi 1985). Thus immunosuppression conditioning has the potential to retard or accelerate disease, depending on the nature of the underlying condition.

Much of the work described thus far has been carried out on laboratory animals. This is not surprising; in order to validate the scientific credibility of a hypothesis it is necessary to perform rigorous and well-controlled scientific experiments. This requires conditions to be standardized with manipulation of a single variable at a time, as well as the use of sufficiently larger numbers of subjects for statistical analyses to be valid. This is all relatively easy in caged laboratory animals and notoriously difficult in human subjects. However, once the hypothesis has been shown to be robust and relevant to the human condition, this warrants investigation in humans. We have already noted how at least one anecdotal report of classical conditioning of the immune system occurred in the literature at the end of the nineteenth century. The rest of this chapter investigates the scientific evidence of such conditioning in humans.

Experimental studies in humans

One study examined the effect of conditioning on the delayed-type hypersensitivity response to tuberculin injection (Smith & McDaniel 1983). A small group of subjects agreed to be given a tuberculin skin test on each arm monthly for 6 months, for which they would be paid $25 per test. Critically, the testing conditions were identical each month: the same office, time and nurse. When they arrived for testing the subjects could see a red vial and a green vial on the desk. The contents of each vial were drawn into a syringe so that the subject could see that the content of the red vial was always applied to the right arm and the content of the green vial to the left arm. Subjects returned to the same office 24 and 48 hours after every administration for the same nurse to assess the extent of reaction to the skin test. In fact the subjects (unbeknown to them) were given an active dose of tuberculin to the right arm and saline to the left arm. This identical protocol was followed for 5 consecutive months but on the 6th month (the experimental trial), without the knowledge of either the nurse or the patient, the content of the vials was switched. Saline was applied to the arm that for the previous 5 months had been given tuberculin and tuberculin was applied to the arm that had previously been given saline. As a control, on the 7th month the subjects were debriefed and a final dose of either tuberculin or saline was administered to the original arm. The results showed that the tuberculin injection caused a stable and measurable reaction for the first 5 weeks whereas the saline injection caused no reaction. However, in the experimental month the arm that was given the tuberculin (the arm that had in previous weeks received saline) showed a very marked reduction in the intensity of its skin reaction. Saline injection to the previously exposed tuberculin arm caused no skin reaction. The following (control) week the reaction to tuberculin was as it had been in the initial 5-month period. Thus, this experiment demonstrated that the delayed hypersensitivity response to tuberculin could be significantly diminished by psychological mediation—that is, the *expectation* that there would be no response in that arm (Smith & McDaniel 1983).

The authors explained their findings in terms of behaviourally conditioned suppression of the immune response. In the experiment the vials, the room, the day of the week and the nurse, as well as the idea that the reactions would always be positive or negative (depending on the arm), served as conditioned stimuli. In fact there were two conditioned responses (one in each arm): the positive response to tuberculin and its associated stimuli, and the negative response to saline with its associated stimuli. The experiment showed that the negative-conditioned response inhibited the unconditioned response to tuberculin whereas the positive-conditioned response did not produce a response to saline.

In the particular paradigm of the above study it was easier to inhibit the unconditioned response than to produce a response in the absence of the unconditioned stimulus. However, more recent experiments have shown that it is possible to produce conditioned enhancement of aspects of immunity using human subjects. Administration of adrenaline, which is capable of causing a transient increase in NK-cell activity, was used as the UCS. After repeated copresentation of the UCS with a neutral CS, re-exposure to the CS alone resulted in a significant increase in NK-cell numbers as well as activity (Buske-Kirschbaum et al 1994). Similarly the immunostimulatory agent interferon gamma (IFN-γ), when used as the UCS paired with a neutral oral CS in a typical classical-conditioning paradigm, induced higher quantifiable levels of cell-mediated immunity in subjects re-exposed to the CS compared with control subjects (Longo et al 1999). These data strongly support the notion that the human immune system can be activated as well as down-regulated by classical conditioning.

Effects in human patients

The experiments so far described indicate that classical conditioning can occur with pairings between inert substances (e.g. neutral drinks) or procedures (e.g. the colour of the vial) and an active agent. The more efficient and rapidly acting the active ingredient the more likely it is that environmental cues or stimuli will be associated with that activity and hence induce a conditioned or 'placebo' response. This suggests that as clinical medicine progresses with the development of sophisticated potent drugs the opportunity for conditioning and the potency of the placebo effect will be dramatically increased. Some very exciting research on the significance of the clinical setting in the treatment of cancer has led the way in this area of research. It has been appreciated for many years that patients repeatedly exposed to nauseating cytotoxic drugs (for chemotherapy) can develop 'anticipatory' nausea prior to drug exposure. As the same cytotoxic drugs are powerful immunosuppressive agents the possibility for anticipatory (or conditioned) immunosuppression presents itself.

In one study, cancer patients previously exposed to three chemotherapy infusions were telephoned to arrange a home assessment at least 3 days before their forthcoming treatment (Bovbjerg et al 1990). In this session psychological tests were administered and a blood sample taken for quantification of cell-mediated immunity. Similar psychological tests and another blood sample was taken from the patients when they next visited the hospital, but before exposure to chemotherapy. The results showed that indices of cell-mediated immunity were lower in the blood sample taken at the hospital compared with the blood collected in the patients' home a few days earlier. Although patients scored higher on measures of anxiety while in the hospital setting this impaired immune response could not be accounted for by anxiety alone. The authors of this study argued that their findings were a consequence of repeated pairing of the hospital stimuli (the CS) with immunosuppressive chemotherapy (the UCS) such that patients showed conditioned immunosuppression in the hospital setting (Bovbjerg et al 1990).

A subsequent and very similar study, however, failed to replicate the finding described above (Fredrikson et al 1993). The discrepancy in the results was explained by subtle differences in procedure between the two studies. In the original study patients arrived at the hospital the night before treatment whereas in the latter study they arrived just a couple of hours prior to treatment. It was hypothesized that conditioned immuno-suppression may occur several hours after exposure to the conditioned stimuli and that the observed effects of the second study represented only the first stage in the treatment setting-induced effect. For example an adrenaline-mediated increase in aspects of immunity may later be followed by the immunosuppressive effect of catecholamines.

CONCLUSION

Examples of conditioned changes in immune function are found in both the humoral and cell-mediated branches of the immune system. Furthermore, aspects of the immune system can be conditioned to be inhibited or enhanced. These conditioned effects are robust and relatively easy to induce, sometimes after just a single pairing with the UCS. The more potent the UCS the easier is the conditioning; this suggests that as more powerful pharmacological agents are developed the potential for conditioning of the immune system within the clinical setting grows. Moreover, patients in a clinical setting may be particularly susceptible to conditioning as they are in a health-deprived state, just as Pavlov's dogs and Ader and Cohen's rats were in a food or water-deprived state. This state of health deprivation makes the individual selectively sensitized to certain health-related cues (e.g. the healer, and associated substances and procedures) and therefore conducive to conditioning. It is not hard therefore to appreciate how the effects observed in the controlled experiments outlined above may substantially contribute to some types of placebo effect. These conditioned responses, though clearly a type of placebo effect, have been shown to be of sufficient physiological magnitude to impact on disease progression. The clinical significance of these findings is only now beginning to be fully appreciated.

REFERENCES

Ader R 1985 Conditioned immunopharmacologic effects in animals: implications for conditioning model of pharmacotherapy. In: White L, Tursky B, Schwartz G (eds) Placebo: theory, research and mechanisms. Guilford, New York, pp 306–323

Ader R, Cohen N 1975 Behaviourally conditioned immunosuppression. Psychosomatic Medicine 37:333–340

Ader R, Cohen N 1982 Behaviourally conditioned immunosuppression and murine systemic lupus erythematosus. Science 215:1534–1536

Ader R, Cohen N 1993 Psychoneuroimmunology: conditioning and stress. Annual Review of Psychology 44:53–85

Alvarez-Borda B, Ramirez-Amaya V, Perez-Montfort R, Bermudez-Rattoni F 1995 Enhancement of antibody production by a learning paradigm. Neurobiology of Learning and Memory 64:103–105

Barnoud P, Le Moal M, Neveu P 1990 Asymmetrical distribution of monoamines in left and right-handed mice. Brain Research 520:317–321

Bovbjerg D H, Redd W H, Maier L A et al 1990 Anticipatory immune suppression and nausea in women receiving cyclic chemotherapy for ovarian cancer. Journal of Consulting and Clinical Psychology 58:153–157

Buske-Kirschbaum A, Kirschbaum C, Stierle H, Jabaij L, Hellhammer D 1994 Conditioned manipulation of natural killer cells in humans using discriminative learning protocol. Biological Psychology 38:143–155

Buske-Kirschbaum A, Grota L, Kirschbaum C et al 1996 Conditioned increases in peripheral blood mononuclear cell (PBMC) number and corticosterone secretion in the rat. Pharmacology, Biochemistry and Behavior 55:27–32

Cechetto D 1993 Experimental cerebral ischaemic lesions and autonomic and cardiac effects in cats and rats. Stroke 24:1–6

Clerici M, Shearer G M 1994 The Th1-Th2 hypothesis of HIV infection: new insights. Immunology Today 15:575–581

Cohen N, Moynihan J A, Ader R 1994 Pavlovian conditioning of the immune system. International Archives of Allergy and Immunology 105:101–106

Davidson R J, Sutton S K 1995 Affective neuroscience: the emergence of a discipline. Current Opinion in Neurobiology 5:217–224

Exton M S, Vo Horsten S, Voge J et al 1998a Conditioned taste aversion produced by cyclosporine A: concomitant reduction in lymphoid organ weight and splenocyte proliferation. Physiology and Behavior 63:241–247

Exton M S, von Horston S, Schult M et al 1998b Behaviourally conditioned immunosuppression using cyclosporine A: central nervous system reduces IL-2 production via splenic innervation. Journal of Neuroimmunology 88:182–191

Fredrikson M, Furst C J, Lekander M, Rotstein S, Blomgren H 1993 Trait anxiety and anticipatory immune reactions in women receiving adjuvant chemotherapy for breast cancer. Brain, Behavior and Immunity 7:79–90

Gainotti G 1969 Reactions 'catastrophiques' et manifestations d'indifference au cours des atteintes cerebrales. Neuropsychologia 7:195–204

Ghanta V K, Demissie S, Hiramoto N S, Hiramoto R N 1996 Conditioning of body temperature and natural killer cell activity with arecoline, a muscarinic cholinergic agonist. Neuroimmunomodulation 3:233–238

Gorczynski R M 1990 Conditioned enhancement of skin allografts in mice. Behavioral Immunity 4:85–92

Gorczynski R M, Kennedy M, Ciampi A 1985 Cimetidine reverses tumour growth enhancement of plasmacytoma tumours in mice demonstrating conditioned immunosuppression. Journal of Immunology 134:4261–4266

Grochowicz P M, Schedlowski M, Husband A J, King M G, Hibberd A D, Bowen K M 1991 Behavioural conditioning prolongs heart allograft survival in rats. Brain, Behavior and Immunity 5:349–356

Gruzelier J, Burgess A, Baldewig T et al 1996 Prospective associations between lateralised brain function and immune status in HIV infection: analysis of EEG, cognition and mood over 30 months. International Journal of Psychophysiology 23:215–224

Hill L E 1930 Philosophy of a biologist. Arnold, London

Kang D-H, Davidson R J, Coe C, Wheeler R E, Tomarken A J, Ershler W B 1991 Frontal brain asymmetry and immune function. Behavioral Neuroscience 105:860–869

Khan A U 1977 Effectiveness of biofeedback and counterconditioning in the treatment of bronchial asthma. Journal of Psychosomatic Research 21:97–104

Klosterhalfen W, Klosterhalfen S 1983 Pavlovian conditioning of immunosuppression modifies adjuvant arthritis in rats. Behavioral Neuroscience 97:663–666

Longo D L, Duffey P L, Kopp W C et al 1999 Conditioned immune response to interferon-gamma in humans. Clinical Immunology 90:173–181

Mackenzie J N 1896 The production of the so called 'rose cold' by means of an artificial rose. American Journal of Medical Science 91:45–57

Martin I 1998 Human electroencephalographic (EEG) response to olfactory stimulation: to experiments using the aroma of food. International Journal of Psychophysiology 30:287–302

Meador K J, Lecuona J M, Helman S W, Loring D W 1999 Differential immunologic effects of language-dominant and non-dominant cerebral resections. Neurology 53:1183–1187

Oppenheimer S, Gelb A, Girvin J, Hachinski V 1992 Cardiovascular effects of human insula cortex stimulation. Neurology 42:1727–1732

Ottenberg P, Stein M, Lewis J, Hamilton C 1958 Learned asthma in the guinea pig. Psychosomatic Medicine 20:395–400

Perez L, Lysle D T 1997 Conditioned immunomodulation: investigations of the role of endogenous activity at mu, kappa and delta opioid receptor subtypes. Journal of Neuroimmunology 79:101–112

Rossi G F, Rosadini G 1967 Experimental analysis of cerebral dominance in man. In: Millikan C H, Danley F L (eds) Brain mechanisms underlying speech and language. Grune & Stratton, New York

Sander D, Klingelhofer J 1995 Changes of circadian blood pressure patterns and cardiovascular parameters indicate lateralisation of sympathetic activation following hemispheric brain infarction. Journal of Neurology 242:313–318

Smith G R, McDaniel P 1983 Psychologically mediated effect on the delayed hypersensitivity reaction to tuberculin in humans. Psychosomatic Medicine 45:65–70

Spector N H, Provinciali M, di Stefano G et al 1994 Immune enhancement by conditioning of senescent mice. Annals of the New York Academy of Sciences 741:283–291

Sullivan R M, Gratton A 1999 Lateralised effects of medial prefrontal cortex lesions on neuroendocrine and autonomic stress responses in rats. Journal of Neuroscience 19:2834–2840

Terzian H 1964 Behavioral and EEG effects of intracarotid sodium amytal injection. Acta Neurochirurgia (Wein) 12:230–239

Tomarken A J, Davidson R J 1994 Frontal brain activation in repressors and non-repressors. Journal of Abnormal Psychology 103:339–349

Tomarken A J, Davidson R J, Wheeler R E, Doss R C 1992 Individual differences in anterior brain asymmetry and fundamental dimensions of emotion. Journal of Personality and Social Psychology 62:676–687

Wheeler R E, Davidson R J, Tomarken A J 1993 Frontal brain asymmetry and emotional reactivity: a biological substrate and affective style. Psychophysiology 30:820–829

Wittling W, Pfluger M 1990 Neuroendocrine hemisphere asymmetries: salivary cortisol secretion during lateralised viewing of emotion-related and neutral films. Brain and Cognition 14:243–265

SECTION 2

Practice

SECTION CONTENTS

Practice

5

How can we optimize non-specific effects?

James Hawkins

Editor's note

James Hawkins presents the therapeutic relationship as the most powerful trigger for self-healing responses. He asks how practitioners can begin to use these effects skillfully. James is an orthopaedic physician, acupuncturist and hypnotherapist. He runs therapy groups and teaches yoga and his particular interest is chronic pain, so in his work he has learned to move fluently between the physical and the psychological aspects of working with pain. He encourages us, however we practice, to take an honest look at how we relate to our clients; and how that shapes the way we work and affects the outcome. More than this he challenges us to take more than just an academic interest in these effects, warning the reader that owning this book is no substitute for action. He explains that though change is difficult, as practitioners we may come to a point where we feel impelled to go beyond just paying lip service to the idea that non-specific effects are significant. Reflection is good, he says, awareness of non-specific effects and their potency is fine, but will you the reader actually do better work with your patients as a result of what you learn from this book? Seeing every consultation as an opportunity to become a clinician-researcher, James argues from the outset that action research can be a conscious way of developing these skills–providing we take care to evaluate their impact rigorously. In this chapter he offers us a took-kit for action research and reflective learning.

> It is not too much science, but a narrow and impoverished view of science, which handicaps contemporary medicine.
>
> *Leon Eisenberg (1988)*

The secret of the care of the patient is in caring for the patient.

Francis Peabody (1927)

...care and Quality are internal and external aspects of the same thing. A person who sees Quality and feels it as he works is a person who cares. A person who cares about what he sees and does is a person who's bound to have some characteristics of Quality.

Robert Pirsig (1974)

THE CHALLENGE

I am writing this chapter because I want to look at some of the practical clinical implications suggested by research on placebo. There is already a wealth of published material highlighting how powerful placebo effects can be. There is also a good deal of fascinating discussion on how we should define the placebo effect and on how it works. I am going to touch only very briefly on these points. This is partly because they are covered at considerable length in other publications (Harrington 1997, White, Tursky & Schwartz 1985) and in other chapters in this book. More importantly it is because I particularly want to explore the personal and practical implications of placebo research. Surprisingly this has not been covered in the literature to anything like the extent that many other aspects of placebo have been. In this chapter I ask: 'What does this research teach me about how to become a better, more helpful, more effective health professional—whatever field I work in?'

Writing style

In my work as a doctor I strive to link my head and my heart. I think medical education often fails trainees in both these areas (Daugherty, Baldwin & Rowley 1998, Eisenberg 1988, Howie 1984, McKegney 1989). I suspect this is true not just for medical education but also for training undergone by those in other branches of the health professions. In writing this chapter I want to experiment with trying to write with both rigour and passion—with both head and heart. Science can be viewed as a methodical way of helping us avoid fooling ourselves. Rigour is important. At the same time I would like to write in a way that is personal and that honours my heart as well. I hope this will do justice to the challenge of taking scientific work on the placebo effect and asking what the implications are for the struggle to become a better therapist. How can this research lead to more helpful therapy for those who, week in, week out, come to the clinic where I work because they are suffering and in pain? Throughout the rest of the chapter I will use the terms 'doctor' and 'therapist' interchangeably. The points made are largely relevant to any health professional.

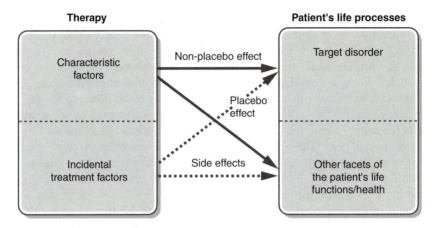

Figure 6.1   Grunbaum's model of placebo effects. (From Grunbaum 1989, with permission.)

DEFINITION, COMPONENTS AND POWER OF THE PLACEBO EFFECT

I think Brody (1997) could be right when he suggests that it might be more sensible at this stage of our knowledge to avoid defining exactly what we mean by the placebo effect. Possibly we should just illustrate the territory we are discussing by giving examples of actual placebo phenomena. Despite this caveat, I do find Grunbaum's model of placebo effects (1989) helpful (see Fig. 6.1). As an academic philosopher, in his writings on placebo he explores precise meanings in considerable detail. He usefully highlights that what is considered a placebo effect or an incidental treatment factor is highly dependent on the overt or covert therapeutic theory that one is using. As research progresses we will hopefully understand more and more about important placebo factors. Holistic therapeutic theories should become better at including these factors as significant aspects of therapeutic interactions. I suggest that what is currently classified as a placebo effect is a marker of our ignorance and the overnarrowness of prevailing therapeutic theory.

Brody (1997), who has great in-depth knowledge of the placebo literature, highlights three important components contributing to a positive placebo response: 'providing an understandable and satisfying explanation of the illness; demonstrating care and concern; and holding out an enhanced promise of mastery or control over the symptoms'. In this chapter I will mainly discuss the third of these components under the general heading of improving expectancy for improvement. However, the practical measures I describe can easily be applied to all three components and I heartily recommend doing this.

As for the power of the placebo effect, I realize that many claims do not stand up to critical examination. Even allowing for this, I think there are still many well-documented cases of powerful placebo responses. Anyone who is familiar with the placebo research field will have their own favourite examples. Studies that fascinate and impress me include the 25% improvement in response rate achieved by being more positive in general practice consultations (Thomas 1987), the great effectiveness of saline injections for severe acute headache pain in an emergency department setting (Harden et al 1996), the finding on meta-analysis that the placebo component of antidepressant medication is nearly twice as powerful as the pharmacological component (Sapirstein 1995), the 70% good or excellent results obtainable when both therapist and patient believe in the effectiveness of placebo interventions (Roberts et al 1993), and the 2.5 times greater death rate over a year's follow-up for postmyocardial infarction patients who took little of their prescribed placebo medication compared with those who took the placebos regularly (Horwitz et al 1990). So where does all this lead us to clinically?

WHAT ARE THE IMPLICATIONS FOR US AS THERAPISTS?

Those who dream by night in the dusty recesses of their minds wake in the day to find it was vanity, but the dreamers of the day are dangerous men for they may act their dream with open eyes to make it possible.

T. E. Lawrence

A useful way to view the process of change

It is not enough simply to know that the placebo effect is a powerful and important aspect of therapeutic encounters. We may know that a particular antibiotic would probably help this patient's chest infection or that relaxation skills would probably help another patient's headaches. Knowing is just the start, however. We then have to explain, prescribe or teach the relevant intervention, monitor its effects and review our own skilfulness in providing this form of help. The transtheoretical stages of change model (Prochaska, DiClemente & Norcross 1992) provides a useful way of viewing many health professionals' relationship to research on the placebo effect. The model highlights five change stages: precontemplation, contemplation, preparation, action and maintenance.

Precontemplation is well described by G. K. Chesterton's remark: 'It isn't that they can't see the solution. It is that they can't see the problem.' Most therapists reading this book on the placebo effect have gone beyond precontemplation. We know that there is a problem. To put it more positively, we know that there are likely to be major therapeutic gains achievable from learning more about what happens in this territory of the placebo effect. Within Prochaska's model we are in the contemplation stage. Contemplators understand that a situation is improvable and are seriously thinking of doing something about it, but they have not made a commitment to take specific action. Unfortunately this shift to specific action does not happen inevitably. The tendency to remain stuck is nicely illustrated by a research study that followed up a group of 200 smokers who had been assessed as being in the contemplation stage in relation to giving up cigarettes (DiClemente & Prochaska 1985, Prochaska & DiClemente 1984). The modal response of the group was to remain in the contemplation stage for the entire 2 years of the project without ever moving to significant action. I suspect this is also true for many health professionals who are sympathetic to learning from placebo research. We are typically so busy that any 'placebo project' is in danger of gathering dust indefinitely.

Does this matter? This is exactly what I would like us to look at just now. Does it matter to us—does it matter to you the reader if your interest in placebo research simply stays as an intellectual interest and no more than that? It would be an awful pity both for us and those who come to us seeking help if in fact there are major lessons to be learnt from this placebo work and yet we never move from contemplation to action. There are possible parallels with a smoker who goes on contemplating stopping cigarettes until one day cancer is diagnosed and the intellectual contemplation is overtaken by brutal reality. We may not be the ones to suffer such consequences but our patients may be. Our patients may suffer very considerably because we never acted on this body of research on placebo although we are all familiar with it. A major objective of this chapter is to provide an opportunity for health professionals to decide whether they want to act rather than just contemplate. Working out what the correct decision is for you personally must surely be worth a few minutes' effort.

A couple of practical exercises

One way of coming at this is to check our priorities. In the end our priorities depend on our values. Here are a couple of brief practical exercises that can be interesting and helpful. The exercises have wide application and I often use one or both for myself or friends or patients when there is a struggle to clarify priorities. It is usually best to use pen and paper but if necessary you can simply think out the responses in your head.

The first method I call the 'respected figures' exercise. Do try it. The initial step is to write down the names of several people who you really respect. Within the context of the placebo effect, it is probably best if you choose figures who you respect in their roles as carers, whether as health professionals or in some other caring role such as voluntary workers, friends or parents. The people you choose can be alive or dead, famous or not, real or fictional, be known personally to you or someone you have only heard about. You do not have to respect everything about them, but in some significant way you respect the way they helped other people. Write down three to six names. Then beside each name write down why you respect this person. What qualities did they show as helpers that you are impressed by? The third step is to group the qualities. Are there some qualities that recur, that several of your respected figures share (even though the qualities may be described in somewhat different words)? The fourth step is to look for the most important qualities, those that recur most often or those that stand out most. Write down the most important or the two or three most important. These are qualities you value very highly. If as a helper of others, you live your life and make your decisions remembering the importance of these qualities, you are likely to feel much more fulfilled and at peace both now and when you come to the end of your life.

The second method to try is the 'eightieth birthday celebration' exercise. It is adapted from the work of Stephen Covey (1989). Imagine that you are 80 years old. People who know and love you have arranged a birthday party. Sit quietly for a little. Imagine that you are at the party feeling warm, happy, fulfilled, glad to be with so many people who care about you and whom you care about. There are several people who are each to say a few words about you. Normally with this exercise one would take people who represented all the different aspects of your life—for example a member of your close family, a good friend, a work colleague, someone from the wider public and so on. In this instance though I suggest you simply take an ex-patient and a work colleague. Each of these two people speaks about you with affection, honesty and respect. They celebrate knowing you and appreciate how you have lived your life, how you have been, what you have done and what you have meant to them. What would you deeply want them to be able to say about you—not now but at your eightieth birthday party when you have lived your life as you would really hope to? Imagine and write down briefly what they said. Take time. Now reread it. How will you need to live your life from now on so that those words will become true? What does this teach you about what your priorities must be? Write the priorities down.

The qualities and priorities that have been highlighted by these two exercises are of central importance for you personally. How do they relate to this issue of placebo research? My reading of the research is that we have underestimated the therapeutic power of caring and of giving hope. Compassion, empathy, reassurance, confidence, kindness—did qualities and priorities like these come up when you did the respected figures and eightieth birthday party exercises? If they did and you want to live an authentic and fulfilling life, surely it is a very high personal priority to move on from contemplation of the placebo research to preparation and action?

What we've seen in our work is that most people don't give themselves permission to live until they've been given a terminal diagnosis.

Stephen Levine (1987)

GOING BEYOND 'JUST THINKING ABOUT IT'

Prochaska and his colleagues have looked both at stages of change and also at processes of change. Change stages describe the *when* of change; change processes describe the *how*. These processes were first identified theoretically by examining recommended change techniques for the leading systems of psychotherapy (Prochaska 1979). Principal component analysis was then used to group the many techniques into a much smaller number of general categories called change processes. At least 10 subsequent principal component analyses conducted on diverse samples and various response formats have yielded similar groupings (Prochaska, DiClemente & Norcross 1992). In total the many change techniques used across hundreds of different forms of psychotherapy can be grouped effectively into just a dozen general change process categories. Box 6.1 lists the 10 process categories that have been reported as receiving most theoretical and empirical research. Definitions and examples of relevant interventions are also listed. Fascinatingly the type of change process that is most helpful seems to vary according to where one is across the five stages of change. This is illustrated in Box 6.2.

To a large extent books like this one on the placebo effect fall within the general change process category of 'consciousness raising'. This process category is appropriate for people who are in the precontemplation and contemplation stages of change. It is likely to be inappropriate and ineffective for those who are moving further through the stages towards actual changes in behaviour. The respected figures and eightieth birthday party exercises we have just used fall under the 'self-re-evaluation' change process category. This type of intervention is usually most helpful for those moving from contemplation to preparation. Prochaska's research categorizes individuals in preparation as those who are intending to take action in the next few weeks. They are involved in decision making and the first stirrings of action. They are ripe to respond to Goethe's injunction: 'Whatever you can do, or dream you can, begin it! Boldness has genius, magic and power in it.'

Box 6.1 The 10 processes of change categories with definitions and examples

Process category	Definition	Intervention examples
Consciousness raising	Increasing information about self and problem	Observations, confrontations, interpretations, bibliotherapy
Self-re-evaluation	Assessing how one feels and thinks about oneself with respect to a problem	Value clarification, imagery, corrective emotional experience
Self-liberation	Choosing and commitment to act or belief in ability to change	Decision-making therapy, New Year's resolutions, logotherapy techniques, commitment-enhancing techniques
Counterconditioning	Substituting alternatives for problem behaviours	Relaxation, desensitization, assertion, positive self-statements
Stimulus control	Avoiding or countering stimuli that elicit problem behaviours	Restructuring one's environment (e.g. removing alcohol or fattening foods), avoiding high-risk cues, fading techniques
Reinforcement management	Rewarding one's self or being rewarded by others for making changes	Contingency contracts, overt and covert reinforcement, self-reward
Helping relationships	Being open and trusting about problems with someone who cares	Therapeutic alliance, social support, self-help groups
Dramatic relief	Experiencing and expressing feelings about one's problems and solutions	Psychodrama, grieving losses, role playing
Environmental re-evaluation	Assessing how one's problem affects physical environment	Empathy training, documentaries
Social liberation	Increasing alternatives for non-problem behaviours available in society	Advocating for rights of repressed, empowering, policy interventions

---

Box 6.1 The five stages of change and associated processes of change categories

Precontemplation	Contemplation	Preparation	Action	Maintenance
Consciousness raising				
Dramatic relief				
Environmental re-evaluation	Self-re-evaluation			
		Self-liberation		
			Reinforcement management	
			Helping relationships	
			Counterconditioning	
			Stimulus control	

From Prochaska, DiClemente & Norcross 1992, with permission.

Problem solving

I am going to assume that you would like to 'begin it', but what exactly should we begin with? How can we best learn from placebo research and move from contemplation through preparation to action and maintenance? The change process category most associated with the move from preparation to action has been labelled 'self-liberation'. It includes the many techniques that involve enhancing belief that one can change, strengthening of commitment and facilitation of decision making. You may already have favourite ways of brainstorming options and coming to a decision. Do go ahead to follow up these approaches. You may also find some of the research on problem solving helpful. A seminal paper, published in the early 1970s, reviewed what was then known about successful problem solving (D'Zurilla & Goldfried 1971). In it the authors commented: 'There has been a remarkable degree of agreement among various theorists and investigators working in different areas as to the general kinds of operations involved in effective problem solving.' This research has been built upon by many subsequent workers (Duckworth 1983, Mynors-Wallis & Gath 1992, Mynors-Wallis et al 1995, Nezu, Nezu & Perri 1989) and clearly highlights the approach as a particularly helpful way of moving from contemplation to action.

Specifics of the problem-solving sequence vary a little from author to author. The approach is based on the common-sense observation that symptoms are typically brought on or aggravated by problems or difficulties. Tackle the problems or difficulties and the symptoms are likely to ease. Symptoms are smoke; problems are fire. Tackle the fire and the smoke will clear. It is also argued that quantifying and monitoring changes in symptoms helps us work out how successful we are being at solving the problems. So the symptoms can be a useful yardstick for measuring progress. For instance, as practitioners we could start with a global symptom like dissatisfaction over the degree to which our clinical practice has improved from our reading of placebo research. This would be interesting. It has been known, however, for many years that successful change is more likely to occur if goals are kept modest and easily measurable (McClelland 1985). Patients' expectancy of improvement and their assessment of the therapeutic alliance are two of the areas highlighted by research as being of key importance in maximizing placebo responses. We now have an opportunity to use problem solving on each of these areas in turn. They are likely to be a rich source of potential clinical applications of placebo research.

How can we encourage expectancy of improvement?

Expectancy-of-improvement scales

In this instance the 'symptom' we want to improve is the patient's expectancy of improvement. Quick, straightforward questionnaires have

Please circle numbers that best describe your reactions to the treatment you are having.

How confident do you feel that this treatment can alleviate your complaint?

   (0 = not at all) **0 1 2 3 4 5 6 7 8 9 10** *(10 = couldn't be more so)*

How confident would you be in recommending this treatment to a friend who suffered from similar complaints?

   (0 = not at all) **0 1 2 3 4 5 6 7 8 9 10** *(10 = couldn't be more so)*

How logical does this treatment seem to you?

   (0 = not at all) **0 1 2 3 4 5 6 7 8 9 10** (10 = couldn't be more so)

Total "attitudes to therapy scale"= sum of three numbers circled above:

Figure 6.2   The attitudes to therapy scale. (From Vincent 1989, with permission.)

been used to assess and monitor patient expectancy. For example Borkovec & Nau (1972) introduced five 10-point expectancy-for-improvement scales and used them to test the credibility of a series of treatment rationales. These scales have been successfully adapted and used by other workers (Petrie & Hazleman 1985, Vincent 1990). The wording of scale questions will vary with the type of treatment being assessed. I give patients a three-question scale that is worded so that it is relevant for most of the treatments I use (see Fig. 6.2).

One possible way into problem solving for better application of placebo research would be to assess your patients' current scores on this scale. Alternatively you could alter the scale questions to reflect the types of treatment used in your own clinical practice. In his research on acupuncture Vincent gave patients the scale to complete after their second and fifth sessions at the clinic. In my own work I typically give out the scale on the same sheet of paper as a scale assessing therapeutic alliance. Appropriate patients may well be asked to complete one or more usually both of these scales after nearly every appointment. I will explain this further in the later discussion on therapeutic alliance.

Identifying problems

The scores on these expectancy-for-improvement scales can now become the 'symptom' we work to improve. The next stage in problem solving involves identifying the problems that are aggravating the symptoms. In this case we are looking for problems or difficulties that are blocking patients from having greater hope and expectancy for improvement. It would be helpful if you, the reader, jotted down a list of such blocks that are relevant for the kinds of patients who you see, the clinical environment that you work in and your own knowledge base, personal state and communication style. The checklist below may suggest additional relevant possibilities:

Patient factors.   These include:

- Lack of knowledge of encouraging aspects of a disease's natural history
- Lack of knowledge of success rates achievable with therapy
- Lack of knowledge of the body–mind's ability to self-heal, adapt and learn
- Previous experience of therapeutic failure
- Depressed mood
- Doubts about the therapist
- Fear of a treatment's side-effects
- Lack of knowledge of what to expect from the treatment and the likely time course necessary
- Lack of knowledge of how to cooperate with the treatment process
- Poor communication.

Clinic environment factors.   These include:

- Appearance and location of clinic
- Appearance and behaviour of staff
- Time constraints and organization of appointments
- Budgetary factors
- The clinic's reputation as a likely source of help
- Optimism and credibility of the person who suggested the clinic visit
- Waiting list size and waiting time at clinic itself.

Therapist factors.   These include:

- Personal appearance of therapist
- Poor history taking and examination
- Poor elicitation of the patient's beliefs, hopes and fears
- Lack of knowledge of encouraging aspects of a disease's natural history
- Lack of knowledge of the range of therapies available, their relative success rates, availability and their advantages and disadvantages
- Lack of familiarity with the treatment chosen, so lack of clarity about what to expect from the treatment, the instructions and warnings to give and the likely time course necessary
- Lack of knowledge of the body–mind's ability to self-heal and adapt
- Pessimism about human beings' abilities to cope and to learn
- Poor communication skills including body language and eye contact
- Unawareness of the importance of giving encouragement

- Poor skills in actually giving specific, convincing encouragement
- Personal stress and burn-out.

From your own insights and with ideas from the checklist, you should be able to construct a problem list. This enumerates factors that you think may be of particular relevance in hindering high levels of expectancy for improvement in the patients that you see. You may want to focus on a subsection of these patients, for example those suffering from a particular disorder or those who do not seem to achieve satisfactory outcomes. Now scan your problem list and select one or two to work on. They should be problems or obstacles that you feel are particularly important or fairly easy to change.

Brainstorming solutions

The next step in problem solving is to brainstorm possible ways of tackling the problems or difficulties that you have selected. When brainstorming allow yourself to be creative and spontaneous. If you are determined to come up with only very good, highly workable solutions you are likely to freeze into producing only a very few, rather constricted ideas. By saving the critical is-this-really-a-good-and-realistic-idea stage till later, you are likely to get a richer mix of options to work with.

As an illustration of the method let us imagine that a therapist came up with the following two problems to tackle. The first is that quite often he does not really believe in the effectiveness of therapies that he suggests to his patients. The second is that he suspects that even when he does believe in the therapy he is using he sometimes fails to share that belief in a genuinely encouraging way with the patient. We know that a therapist's confidence in the therapy used is important and can leak across to the patient even in single-blind research studies (Gracely et al 1985, LeRoy 1941). Similarly, actively encouraging patients that they are likely to bene-fit from therapy and get better adds considerably to the effectiveness of therapeutic interventions (Thomas 1987).

Brainstorming the first problem of lack of belief, here are 10 possible solutions that I came up with in just under 7 minutes (I did go back to tidy up the wording): (1) make sure that for the common problems that patients present to me I am up to date with what interventions are considered optimal from current research (Haynes et al 1986); (2) set aside a regular time to go into the library each week; (3) explore what journals I can scan on the internet; (4) join or set up a journal club; (5) ask the advice of respected colleagues about how best to keep up to date; (6) subscribe to evidence-based medicine journals that scan and abstract from a wide range of publications; (7) challenge myself to give a lecture or write a short article about any particularly thorny types of problem;

(8) record over a few clinics which types of patient or problem most regularly trouble me with this feeling of lack of therapeutic belief; (9) take trouble to construct a list of those whom I can refer difficult problems to when I feel outside my areas of expertise; (10) ask myself what I would want to do if specific difficult problems happened to me or to someone I loved.

Similarly one can brainstorm for responses to the suspicion that even when one does believe in the therapy one is using sometimes there may be a failure to share that belief in a really encouraging way with the patient. I came up with the following 10 ideas. Again this took between 6 and 7 minutes (plus some time for tidying up the wording): (1) using a sheet of paper with the initials or numbers of the patients I see during a clinic, record on a 0–10 scale after each consultation how encouraging I really felt I was (0 = not at all encouraging; 10 = as appropriately encouraging as I could possibly be); (2) tape record a series of consultations and listen to the recordings to assess the degree of encouragement I gave using a similar scale; (3) ask patients to fill in a version of the attitudes to therapy scale and compare the answers with a similar therapist's scale that I have filled in myself; (4) find a colleague who would be interested to explore this issue with me and go over the results of these explorations together; (5) work out what each of us did well or badly and make explicit intentions how each of us wants to change—then later review together how well we did; (6) go to a course on non-directive hypnotherapy and see whether ideas about suggestions given outside formal trance are of interest; (7) think hard about non-verbal aspects of reassurance such as voice tone, body position, touch, gaze and so on; (8) explore the possible use of video; (9) ask about and read literature on relevant aspects of the consultation; (10) use written and taped material as hand-outs to underline reassuring points to patients.

So much for examples: to make this relevant and useful for yourself and your patients, take just 5 to 10 minutes and brainstorm possible responses to one of the problems you selected. Remember that you do not have to be too sensible or realistic at this stage. Now go over the ideas you came up with and see whether there are any that you would like to try out. This is the point where more realism needs to come in. You may find on rereading that you want to adapt one of the initial ideas or combine two or more ideas into something more appropriate.

Action and maintenance

We are now moving into what Prochaska, DiClemente & Norcross (1992) define as the action and maintenance stages of change. These authors suggest that particularly helpful change process categories for these two change stages are: helping relationships (e.g. involving interested colleagues), counterconditioning (e.g. writing down a succinct statement of what you intend to do and why it is important to you), stimulus control (e.g. making sure that you are not too rushed to try out your ideas by keeping your intentions realistic and scheduling in adequate time) and reinforcement management (e.g. acknowledging that making these kinds of changes requires determination and persistence). Work out a reward system for yourself and experiment to see if it encourages you to keep going with your intentions. The time management and behavioural literatures recommend similar kinds of techniques.

For intentions to be effective:

• Make sure that the intentions make good sense to you and that you really want to achieve them.

• Check that the intentions are realistically achievable in the time you have available.

• Write the intentions down in a concrete specific form. This means it should be very clear whether you have achieved them or not. For example 'read more research' is not adequate as an intention. 'Spend at least half an hour weekly reading relevant articles from the British Medical Journal and keep a record of the time spent', is adequately concrete and specific.

• Be clear about the time periods involved. When are you going to start and how long will you continue for before you review the value of the intentions?

• How will you assess whether the intentions have been useful or not?

• Work out when during the week you are going to make time for the intention and write it clearly into your diary as high priority.

• If possible involve another person or persons and make sure that everyone has written records of what specific intentions have been made and when they are to be checked.

This kind of approach can help us go beyond 'just thinking about it'. It is important to be realistic too. Good intentions tend to decay over time. Evolving scientific research in our fields of interest and the continuing education seminars available to us tend repeatedly to emphasize the 'what' of medicine rather than the 'how'. Additionally the pressures and demands on our time that we face every week tend as well to erode our intentions to practise medicine in more holistic ways. This is the reality for most of us. The literature on getting free from addictions shows a similar pattern. The stages of change—precontemplation, contemplation, preparation, action and maintenance—often move in a spiral. That is OK: if we are swimming across a lake and know there is a steady cross-current pushing us sideways off our course, we just have to correct for the cross-current. It is the same in our lives as health professionals. The culture pushes us sideways so we tend to become just rushed technicians rather than healers and practitioners of whole person medicine. Writing regular reminders in our diaries, involving others in support groups and reading literature that reminds us of the importance of working from our hearts as well as our heads are just some ways of helping to counteract the cultural cross current. Guarding against the tendency to slip back into old ways can become a useful problem-solving exercise in its own right.

WARMTH, INTEREST, EMPATHY AND CARING

The way is not in the sky. The way is in the heart.

Dhammapada

How can patients feel more listened to and cared for?

Much of what has been said about encouraging a patient's expectancy for improvement can also be applied to the at least equally important area of helping patients feel listened to and cared for. Brody (1997) in his thoughtful writing on 'the doctor as therapeutic agent' emphasizes this fact. When asked to describe the qualities that make a good doctor, patients list attributes such as kindness, willingness to listen, sympathy, patience, tolerance and understanding (Sachs 1982). It is these qualities that are associated with greater patient satisfaction (Cape 1996, Silove, Parker & Manicavasagar 1990). A good therapeutic alliance, however, does not just improve patient satisfaction: it also improves therapeutic outcome, both for psychotherapy (Blatt et al 1996, Burns & Auerbach 1996, Horvath & Symonds 1991) and for pharmacotherapy (Krupnick et al 1996, Weiss et al 1997). This latter finding seems less surprising in the light of a recent meta-analysis of placebo antidepressant research by Sapirstein (1995). The data indicated that 23% of the response to antidepressant medication was due to spontaneous remission, 27% to the drug and 50% to the placebo effect. An earlier meta-analysis suggested an even more powerful role for placebo antidepressants (Greenberg et al 1992).

We have already discussed how to move from merely contemplating the importance of bettering patients' expectancies for improvement to specific action plans involving changes in clinical practice. The exercises we have done on respected figures and the eightieth birthday party are likely also to have thrown up priorities in this further area of the therapist's kindness, patience, tolerance and understanding. It makes very good sense therefore to redo the problem-solving exercise or some similar technique to clarify what changes you might want to make in moving from the contemplation stage to action and maintenance in this area as well. We earlier discussed the use of quick, straightforward questionnaires for assessing and monitoring patient expectancy. There are many more instruments available for monitoring general therapeutic alliance. I personally have benefited from reviewing my practice with the brief patient satisfaction questionnaire

Put a tick (✓) in the box to the right to indicate how strongly you agree with each of the following 10 statements about how you experienced the most recent appointment with your doctor	0 = not at all	1 = somewhat	2 = moderately	3 = a lot
1.	I felt that I could trust my doctor during today's session				
2.	My doctor felt I was worthwhile				
3.	My doctor was friendly and warm towards me				
4.	My doctor understood what I said during today's session				
5.	My doctor was sympathetic and concerned about me				
Add scores for items 1-5					
6.	Sometimes my doctor did not seem to be completely genuine				
7.	My doctor pretended to like me more than he or she really does				
8.	My doctor did not always seem to care about me				
9.	My doctor did no always understand the way I felt inside				
10	My doctor acted condescendingly and talked down to me				
Add scores for items 6-10					

Figure 6.3 The empathy scale. (From Burns & Auerbach 1996, with permission.)

developed by Cope and colleagues (Cope et al 1986). For psychotherapy patients I now fairly routinely use Burns' therapeutic empathy scale (Fig. 6.3). Burns makes great claims for the value of using such scales and his careful research suggests that he has a valid point. As he puts it: 'The use of the ES (empathy scale) … on a trial basis with even a few patients will usually convince the skeptical therapist that these instruments cannot only be useful but can have a revolutionary effect on one's practice, regardless of the therapist's orientation' (Burns & Auerbach 1996).

In some ways there are even more compelling reasons for attending to health professionals' empathy, warmth and respect than there are for improving patient expectancy. Research shows that feelings of warmth and compassion can have immediate beneficial effects on the well-being of therapists themselves (Rein, Atkinson & McCraty 1995). This contrasts with the personal cost in physical symptoms, immunological status and psychological upset caused by feelings of frustration and anger. Over the longer term, cynicism and hostility can have more permanently devastating consequences. Barefoot, Dahlstrom & Williams (1983) followed up 255 medical graduates for 25 years. They found that the 119 with hostility scores greater than the median had six times the death rate of the 136 who scored at or less than the median. The families of health professionals can be caught in this fall-out too. There is little information available but Sakinofsky (1980) compared suicide rates amongst the wives of men in a dozen different occupations in England and Wales. Doctors' wives killed themselves much more frequently than the wives of any of the other groups. Gabbard and coworkers (Gabbard, Menninger & Coyne 1987) found no relationship between longer hours and turmoil in medical marriages. Complaint of insufficient time appeared to be more an excuse for marital discord than an explanation. Wives were most upset by their doctor husbands' lack of emotional intimacy, conversation, empathy and respect.

It is not just the placebo effect that demands health professionals should attend more to our capacity to show warmth, empathy and compassion. It seems the warning that such open-heartedness will speed burn-out may be the opposite of what actually occurs. For the sake of our own well-being, our life expectancy, the health of those closest to us and our helpfulness as health workers it is immensely important that we move from contemplation to action. The problem-solving methods already discussed can highlight where we can start. Possibilities include looking after our own health better—improved health tends to lead to better mood and less hostility and frustration (Nouri & Beer 1989), working on our own personal blocks (Curtis et al 1995, Firth-Cozens 1992), more effective time management, longer appointment times (Howie, Porter & Forbes 1989), better continuity of patient care (Hjortdahl & Laerum 1992, Schmittdiel et al 1997), training in communication skills and more regular feedback from patient questionnaires (Delbanco 1996). Qualitative research with nurses (Montgomery 1996) chosen by their peers as 'exemplars' of caring highlights a less discussed area. It seems that it is not just the closeness of a helping relationship that matters, it is also the quality of that closeness. Allowing compassion and empathy without burning out too easily may involve a sense of common humanity, of going beyond the ego. As one caregiver put it: 'Our clients are a part of our heart, and helping to heal them heals our hearts as well.' This resonates with the beautiful words of Albert Einstein: 'A human being is a part of the whole, called by us the "Universe", a part limited in time and space. He experiences himself, his thoughts and feelings, as something separated from the rest—a kind of optical delusion of his consciousness. The delusion is a kind of prison for us, restricting us to our personal desires and to affection for a few persons nearest to us. Our task must be to free ourselves from this prison by widening the circle of compassion to embrace all living creatures and the whole of nature in its beauty. Nobody is able to achieve this completely, but the striving for such achievement is in itself a part of the liberation and a foundation for inner security.'

REFERENCES

Barefoot J C, Dahlstrom W G, Williams R B 1983 Hostility, CHD incidence, and total mortality: a 25-year follow-up study of 255 physicians. Psychosomatic Medicine 45:59–63

Blatt S J, Zuroff D C, Quinlan D M, Pilkonis P A 1996 Interpersonal factors in brief treatment of depression: further analyses of the National Institute of Mental Health Treatment of Depression Collaborative Research Project. Journal of Consulting and Clinical Psychology 64:162–171

Borkovec T D, Nau S D 1972 Credibility of analogue therapy rationales. Journal of Behavior Therapy and Experimental Psychiatry 3:257–260

Brody H 1997 The doctor as therapeutic agent: a placebo effect research agenda. In: Harrington A (ed) The placebo effect: an interdisciplinary exploration. Harvard University Press, Cambridge, MA

Burns D D, Auerbach A 1996 Therapeutic empathy in cognitive-behavioral therapy: does it really make a difference? In: Salkovskis P (ed) Frontiers of cognitive therapy. Guilford Press, New York, p 147

Cape J D 1996 Psychological treatment of emotional problems by general practitioners. British Journal of Medical Psychology 69:85–99

Chesterton G K

Cope D W, Linn L S, Leake B D, Barrett P A 1986 Modification of residents' behavior by preceptor feedback of patient satisfaction. Journal of General Internal Medicine 1:394–398

Covey S R 1989 The seven habits of highly effective people. Simon & Schuster, London

Curtis K A, Davis C M, Trimble T K, Papoulidis D K 1995 Early family experiences and helping behaviors of physical therapists. Physical Therapy 75:1089–1100

Daugherty S R, Baldwin D C, Rowley B D 1998 Learning, satisfaction, and mistreatment during medical internship: a national survey of working conditions. Journal of the American Medical Association 279:1194–1199

Delbanco T L 1996 Quality of care through the patient's eyes. British Medical Journal 313:832–833

DiClemente C C, Prochaska J O 1985 Processes and stages of change: coping and competence in smoking behavior change. In: Schiffman S, Wills T A (eds) Coping and substance abuse. Academic Press, San Diego, CA, pp 319–343

Duckworth D H 1983 Evaluation of a programme for increasing the effectiveness of personal problem-solving. British Journal of Psychology 74:119–127

D'Zurilla T J, Goldfried M R 1971 Problem solving and behavior modification. Journal of Abnormal Psychology 78:107–126

Eisenberg L 1988 Is there too much science in medicine or not enough? Advances 4(4):18–28

Firth-Cozens J 1992 The role of early family experience in the perception of organizational stress: fusing clinical and organizational perspectives. Journal of Occupational and Organizational Psychology 65:61–75

Gabbard G O, Menninger R W, Coyne L 1987 Sources of conflict in medical marriages. American Journal of Psychiatry 144:567–572

Goethe J W von

Gracely R H, Dubner R, Deeter W R, Wolskee P J 1985 Clinicians' expectations influence placebo analgesia. Lancet i:43

Greenberg R P, Bornstein R F, Greenberg M D, Fisher S 1992 A meta-analysis of antidepressant outcome under 'blinder' conditions. Journal of Consulting and Clinical Psychology 60:664–669

Grunbaum A 1989 The placebo concept in medicine and psychiatry. In: Shepherd M, Sartorius N (eds) Non specific aspects of treatment. Hans Huber, Toronto, p 12

Harden R N, Gracely R H, Carter T, Warner G 1996 The placebo effect in acute headache management: ketorolac, meperidine, and saline in the emergency department. Headache 36:352–356

Harrington A (ed) 1997 The placebo effect: an interdisciplinary exploration. Harvard University Press, Cambridge, MA

Haynes R B, McKibbon K A, Fizgerald D, Guyatt G H, Walker C J, Sackett D L 1986 How to keep up with the medical literature. I–VI. Annals of Internal Medicine 105:149–153, 309–312, 474–478, 636–640, 810–824, 978–984

Hjortdahl P, Laerum E 1992 Continuity of care in general practice: effect on patient satisfaction. British Medical Journal 304:1287–1290

Horvath A O, Symonds B D 1991 Relation between working alliance and outcome in psychotherapy: a meta-analysis. Journal of Counseling Psychology 38:139–149

Horwitz R I, Viscoli C M, Berkman L et al 1990 Treatment adherence and risk of death after a myocardial infarction. Lancet 336:542–545

Howie J G R 1984 Research in general practice: pursuit of knowledge or defence of wisdom? British Medical Journal 288:1507–1511

Howie J G R, Porter A M D, Forbes J F 1989 Quality and the use of time in general practice: widening the discussion. British Medical Journal 298:1008–1010

Kaufman G 1997 Placebo: conversations at the disciplinary borders. In: Harrington A (ed) The placebo effect: an interdisciplinary exploration. Harvard University Press, Cambridge, MA, p 243

Krupnick J L, Sotsky S M, Simmens S et al 1996 The role of the therapeutic alliance in psychotherapy and pharmacotherapy outcome: findings in the National Institute of Mental Health Treatment of Depression Collaborative Research Program. Journal of Consulting and Clinical Psychology 64:532–539

LeRoy G V 1941 The effectiveness of the xanthine drugs in the treatment of angina pectoris. Journal of American Medical Association 116:921–925

Levine S 1987 Healing into life and death. Gateway Books, Bath

McClelland D C 1985 Human motivation. Scott, Foresman, Glenview, IL

McKegney C P 1989 Medical education: a neglectful and abusive family system. Family Medicine 21:452–457

Montgomery C L 1996 The care-giving relationship: paradoxical and transcendant aspects. Alternative Therapies 2(2):52–57

Mynors-Wallis L M, Gath D H 1992 Brief psychological treatments. International Review of Psychiatry 4:301–306

Mynors-Wallis L M, Gath D H, Lloyd-Thomas A R, Tomlinson D 1995 Randomised controlled trial comparing problem solving treatment with amitriptyline and placebo for major depression in primary care. British Medical Journal 310:441–445

Nezu A M, Nezu C M, Perri M G 1989 Problem-solving therapy for depression: theory, research and clinical guidelines. John Wiley, New York

Nouri S, Beer J 1989 Relations of moderate physical exercise to scores on hostility, aggression, and trait-anxiety. Perceptual and Motor Skills 68:1191–1194

Peabody F W 1927 The care of the patient. Journal of the American Medical Association 88:877–882

Petrie J, Hazleman B 1985 Credibility of placebo transcutaneous nerve stimulation and acupuncture. Clinical and Experimental Rheumatology 3:151–153

Pirsig R M 1976 Zen and the art of motorcycle maintenance: an inquiry into values. Corgi, London

Prochaska J O 1979 Systems of psychotherapy: a transtheoretical analysis. Dorsey, Homewood, IL

Prochaska J O, DiClemente C C 1984 The transtheoretical approach: crossing traditional boundaries of change. Dorsey, Homewood, IL

Prochaska J O, DiClemente C C, Norcross J C 1992 In search of how people change. American Psychologist 47:1102–1114

Rein G, Atkinson M, McCraty R 1995 The physiological and psychological effects of compassion and anger. Journal of Advancement in Medicine 8(2):87–105

Roberts A H, Kewman D G, Mercier L, Hovell M 1993 The power of nonspecific effects in healing. Clinical Psychology Review 13:375–391

Sachs H 1982 Can patients influence health decisions? Journal of the Royal College of General Practitioners 32:691–694

Sakinofsky I 1980 Suicide in doctors and wives of doctors. Canadian Family Physician 26:837–844

Sapirstein G 1995 The effectiveness of placebos in the treatment of depression: a meta-analysis. Doctoral dissertation, University of Connecticut, Storrs, CT

Schmittdiel J, Selby J V, Grumbach K, Quesenberry C P 1997 Choice of a personal physician and patient satisfaction in a health maintenance organization. Journal of the American Medical Association 278:1596–1599

Silove D, Parker G, Manicavasagar V 1990 Perceptions of general and specific therapist behaviors. Journal of Nervous and Mental Disease 178:292–299

Thomas K B 1987 General practice consultations: is there any point in being positive? British Medical Journal 294:1200–1202

Vincent C A 1989 A controlled trial of the treatment of pain by acupuncture. Clinical Journal of Pain 5:305–312

Vincent C 1990 Credibility assessment in trials of acupuncture. Complimentary Medical Research 4(1):8–11

Weiss M, Gaston L, Propst A, Wisebord S, Zicherman V 1997 The role of the alliance in the pharmacologic treatment of depression. Journal of Clinical Psychiatry 58:196–204

White L, Tursky B, Schwartz G E (eds) 1985 Placebo: theory, research, and mechanisms. Guilford, New York

6

Some reflections on creating therapeutic consultations*

David Reilly

Lecture	Questions from the floor

Editor's note

David Reilly is a physician, a homeopath and hypnotherapist. He is also a leading medical innovator as well as a researcher and a teacher of holistic health care. In this chapter David reminds us that medicine mirrors the culture that spawns it; and in our society the mind–body split is a deep and tenacious assumption. Science deals with what is tangible and measurable and nowhere is its everyday impact on how we see ourselves greater than in medicine. But modern medicine, cautions Reilly, has become so terribly focused on the technical that a patient's humanity and the practitioner's character have disappeared from the equation, leaving only the medication and the disease. With reference to the placebo effect, for 'real' medicine, human-to-human aspects are ephemeral or worse, fraudulent. This notion, as it seeped into medical thinking and education, encouraged a culture that Reilly believes has been destructive or doctors' capacity to care. He wants to change that and here he tells us how. But he also warns that de-humanising processes can happen wherever purely technical aspects or practice are over-valued at the expense of the art of healing. Reilly says complementary therapies are not spared this danger and he unfolds a landscape where the therapeutic relationship can live alongside technical expertise. Giving us a glimpse into his own way of working with humour and language, he puts over a deeper message about the therapeutic power of compassion and empathy.

LECTURE

As I understand it, life is not yet understood. Indeed, it may even be a placebo response for all I know. It might not even be understandable, if I could radically put to us, by our minds. Because we do have limits. I've never met an ant with a PhD, for example, and there are no chimpanzees in this audience. Undoubtedly the life forms that we are sets limits. It may

This chapter is taken from a transcript of Dr Reilly's lecture with minimum editing leaving it in the reflective style of the talk.

indeed be that we were not clever enough to put our own hearts into our chests or the Sun in the sky. Nevertheless, we are life, and the fact that it may be beyond our understanding doesn't mean to say that we can't work with it. We are conscious within life, and we can learn to live in the jungle, as it were.

Perhaps the term 'placebo' is one window on aspects of life in action—but really the issue is life. Life has an innate tendency to heal and come to order as well as a tendency to destroy. Recently the latter has been given the term 'apoptosis', which is programmed cell death, and seems to be built into life, into its substance. These tendencies are the essence of it, as I see it, and we influence these tendencies, forming a relationship with life.

This relationship with life in a healing context is as old as we are, and parents and loved ones have been part of that throughout time. It's undoubtedly full of wonders, some of which I would like to touch on in a way that I hope will be complementary to the other speakers.

I think shamanism for tens of thousands of years has been looking at this issue of life in action and life in healing. At times, within the relationship with life in a healing context, I'm now confident that transformation is possible—catalysing the built-in healing potential within ourselves, within our patients. Sometimes the transformation is of physical processes or physical healing. Sometimes the transformation is more in our relationship with the process of life and of being unwell—and that indeed may be the more important transformation given our frailty and given our mortality.

I'll call this transformation 'healing', and we could speak of it in a medical context as being a therapeutic change or therapeutic effect. For some years I've been quietly trying to suggest that the term placebo be renamed in some way, perhaps in relation to the self-healing response. Recently I've been toying around with other words, maybe something like 'intention-modified healing responses'. I quite like that one because it abbreviates to I-MOHRE, suggesting in the pun the consciousness of I and its impact with the encounter. Of course that can then also interreact with specific therapies and their specific effects, and that that would abbreviate to TIMOHRE 'therapy- and intention-modified self-healing'—a tying together of these elements.

In wandering down these paths I'm aware there are many people here who could give the talk that I'm giving, and that many of you have more wisdom in this area. I'm really just acting as a voice for our understanding and a backdrop to our thoughts. Perhaps the conclusion is that these elements, of healing, of transformation and of working with life, have to a degree been sidelined in medical care, even despised. Sometimes parts of it have been placed under the term 'placebo'. I think a lot of wisdom lies buried under that 'X' on the map, and I see our job now is to excavate those gems and bring them back to the work that unites us all, which is trying to become more skilled in working this relationship, in these therapeutic encounters. Dr Benson has given you a feel from the scientific literature of some of the sorts of work and experimental results in this area so my chat will not be a literature review, more a wandering or a reflection. The wandering is in search of therapeutic encounters, looking forward to the idea that therapeutic work and encounters might once more find their place at the heart of medicine and the heart of caring. Then the concept of placebo would to an extent then become redundant; we would simply be examining those factors that successfully affect healing encounters.

I'd like to start our search for this wisdom with ourselves—before we became carers, as patients, because most of us have been or will be patients at some stage—this is something that unites us. But even before we were patients we had often more understanding about healing and healing encounters that we would subsequently learn in our professional training.

Think of your own responses, of how you would like a loved one cared for—someone very close to you who's threatened perhaps by some significant disease or possibility of an impact in their life. In that circumstance you know already what to do, you know those feelings, you know those instincts, and that's before we've even begun our training. So we all know what healing feels like and what's good and isn't good in these encounters. Someone once said: 'What do you get when you analyse a glass of water? I don't know, but it's nothing you can drink.' And roughly we all know when we've been hit in some way, and we all know when we've received a truly tender kiss in some way. When a child is in distress we know what to do, and we know what to do to make a difference. These basic understandings are there before they became complicated with words like autonomic nervous system, and psychoneuroimmunology, and placebo and nocebo and the subconscious, and the various words and terms that we then use to begin to get to grips with this simple in-built understanding. The transition into professional life of that knowledge is where a lot of our problems are developing. I remember a teacher telling me that there was a study that you might be aware of, which suggested that at the point of entry into medical school—this was in Germany I believe—the students were noted to have above-average caring attitudes, and at the point of exit they had become below average. Something's happening—and I'd like to talk a wee bit about some of that.

I think many of us in our professional studies began to drift away from this basic understanding when we met our first patient—because for many of us our first patient was a dead one. Then we proceeded to cut them up. Something gets brutalized in our induction into our healing work and we lose it. I recall the sense of sanctity of the medical students around the corpse on the first day, standing in silence as it was draped in white. I wouldn't want to tell you the things that occurred on the last day, and for those of you that haven't been around it you would find it disturbing.

There had clearly been an induction process, there had clearly been a brutalizing and there had clearly been a potential loss of respect.

Then as we continue in our training we learn that a significant part of our job is to stop things happening. I'd like you to look at this slide with a fresh eye if you would; this is a major drug company's vision to take our future development of our medicines, and five marks for anyone that can spot a common theme. [Laughter. The slide shows a research campaign for new drugs—every one begins with 'anti' as in antihistamine, antidepressant and so on.] Now, the thing is, sometimes when you're up so close to something you don't know it any more, you don't see it any more; it becomes a background noise. But indeed there is a dominant thought process behind many of the forms of orthodox training that I was induced into. The idea is that the wisdom lies within us, the professional; we understand what's wrong and we step in and block a reaction in the patient in some way. This is good, and I use this sort of care all the time. However, there is a balance point; there is a slide that could have every word on it begin with 'pro', for example, which would be something to do with bringing out the potential inherent in living organisms and within human beings, and stimulating and encouraging that potential. I think some of that wisdom is again buried under the term 'placebo'.

As I sought some understanding I had many people who inspired me. I recall one consultant who taught me a great deal. He took us as a group of medical students to see a lady in the acute receiving ward. We marched up to the bed; without introduction or words he ripped the bedclothes back to reveal her breasts, and then proceeded to express milk from the breast saying 'you see, this lady has a prolactinoma' (a brain tumour making hormones), and I recall that man now, and he's a good man, doing good work and doing the best that he can. But he helped me see this wasn't right. He helped me see that something was going fundamentally wrong in our healing encounters and in our system of care.

I'd like to thank the obstetrical sister, 24 going on 44, who caused me to walk out on my obstetrical training. 'Fathers' she said 'shall be allowed in the room when Sister says so. Father shall stand at the head of the bed. Father shall take mother's hand. Father shall leave the room when doctor enters.' Meantime there was the lady lying on her back giving birth, bright fluorescent lights, the doors bursting open as the doctor came in to put a fetal electrode on her baby's scalp. She thought it was for the baby's welfare; it was in fact a piece of research that the registrar was doing. Then I had my own experience as a patient, and you've all had that too, when you know that the water isn't good enough to drink in some way, that there's something not right in the water.

Then you leave the beginnings of this professional induction and you join what is after all a culture. It's important to remember as human beings we're within that culture. There can be lots of individuality within it, and there can be a way of doing things because we're people. I remember taking 4th-year medical students; it was the first time that I was teaching them their orthodox medicine at the Royal Infirmary in Glasgow. We were round the bed of a lady and we sat down and I said to the first student at the foot of the bed 'Would you like to take this lady's history?' She began 'What age are you?' I said: 'Stop! Why did you ask that? What do you do when you meet someone?' 'Well I introduce myself.' I said 'Have you not just met someone?' 'Oh, am I supposed to do that?'

The next term I had to teach 3rd-year students who had never seen a patient, at least a live one. I decided before I'd let them loose to send one of them out of the room and asked her to come back in and take my history. I swear to God, she walked in the room, didn't look me in the eye, sat down and said 'What age are you?' I said 'Why? Why are you talking to me like that? What are you saying?' and then all of a sudden I had a change in my perception, like a little image, I suddenly saw the students sitting round me and they were 7 years old and their legs weren't touching the ground, and I realize they were very, very frightened indeed. So without announcement I turned to the first student and I said 'Hello, I understand your name is (I made up a name) and you were admitted last night as an emergency; would you like to tell me what happened?' Now, very quickly the student engaged, didn't quite understand but engaged, and began to tell me a story about how she had been admitted last night from what in fact was a drug overdose. Then I turned to the next person at the table and said 'As her brother, how have you been feeling about that, what's happening with you?' Then we went round the table and eventually I brought the atmosphere down gently and back to a more normal state of mind.

I was able to say to them: 'That is what's called a consultation'. A consultation is if you like when the room disappears; that's quite a good check on a consultation. Like any good encounter, it's like looking in the face of a friend during a serious or important discussion. You know, those students just took off, they went into the wards, they shook hands, they said hello, they asked people how they were, they sat down spontaneously on the bedside, just because I'd given them permission. I'd said to them: 'Look, you haven't come here as a blank page, you've come here having cried and laughed and been frightened and loved and hated, and being in families and being in life. And you've come here to develop this in some way. Not to learn from scratch.' These students explained to me that they had had their core communication skills training already. [Laughter.] Okay, and this could be part of the problem—professionalization. They explained to me that they were taken into rooms for mock consultations with video cameras set up and they said they very quickly picked up the understanding that the teachers were 'the experts'. 'You don't know; we know; we're going to tell you how to communicate. This is an open question; this is a closed question; this is this thing; this is that thing.' Their basic pretraining instincts, their humanness, wasn't being valued in some way and wasn't being championed. I think this is part of the mental state that's capable of taking some of these elements and calling them placebo responses further down the line in our medical and scientific enquiry.

Then you learn words and distinctions like organic versus functional, and somewhere in between that, and you're not quite sure what they mean, you learn the word placebo in the passing. Now placebo's a bit of an odd word. You've got this definite feeling it's something to do with psychiatry or that side of life. There's maybe something a bit unsavoury about it. It may be linked to Bedlam in some way. I remember doing a seminar with some final-year students and they were telling about a man who'd come in the night before with chest pain, and someone had wondered did he have 'real' chest pain. So they injected him with saline and the chest pain settled. This was the cue for the students to laugh. It's an interesting reaction. I said 'so let's talk a wee bit about that' and we wandered into an area that brought us up into discussion of so-called alternative medicine, and a student gave me a time-honoured quote:

Oh
isn't
it
just
a
placebo
response?

I've printed it this way because it tells us so much:

'Oh'—the emotional tone that surrounds this subject
'Isn't——the preconception.
'It'—the idea that it's just one thing.
'Just'—the diminutive, what does it matter anyway.
'Placebo response'——singular.

So I asked him what training he'd had on placebo responses or healing, and he said none. That's when I realized that medical training reaches the part that the mind hasn't yet examined.

This attitude is interesting because it turns out that medical students are maybe more responsive to placebo than average. I don't know if you know where this advert came from. [Slide: two cartoon faces, the eyes are red tablets (of an antidepressant) and the caption reads 'Have you seen the red effect, the red effect in depression?'] From the The Lancet in the mid 1970s, a study of 300 medical students given placebos or psychotropic (mind-altering) drugs—some were downers and some were uppers. About 50% of the students showed clear psychological changes and 60% showed physical changes. They correctly identified the red tablets as the stimulants, and the blue tablets as the depressants. The interesting thing is that every tablet was a placebo—in all 300 instances (Blackwell, Bloomfield & Burcher 1972). Now, sometimes the microcosm manufactures the macrocosm as they say; even within that tiny slide and that tiny story lies I think some very important lessons in the fact, for example, that our healing systems can be activated by the subtlety of symbolism, of even just colour. There are many such stories in the placebo literature of these effects.

A core dilemma is the issue of 'organic' ('real/physical') versus 'functional' (no tissue changes); this mind/body distinction, which is so inherent in our training, is enough to make you blush—and I choose my example carefully. I think blushing is quite important actually, because again without a medical degree, or perhaps especially if you haven't got one, you realize that blushing reflects the unity of our mind and body experience. We could take thermograms and neurotransmitter profiles and lab it up in all sorts of ways with changes in hormones and blood flow during a blush. These changes occur in a moment, and why? Because of our inner world, because of our feelings. This closeness, this intimacy that lies there is actually inherently obvious to us if we just step back a little and reflect on it. It is very important; I believe it often impacts on whether we will get unwell and to what degree we might recover. The main aspect of therapeutic encounters may be working the interfaces, the gaps, between our inner and our outer worlds, between our conscious and our subconscious and between our inner world and our physical system.

Then, as we head off as more matured carers, perhaps a principal driving force is peer determination. After a while it becomes pretty automatic, a bit like driving. If it wasn't in the curriculum it's definitely not true, and if it's not in the sacred text of the Lancet and the British Medical Journal it most certainly isn't true. It gets easier when you realize that medicine and religion came from the same root, and that these bibles are the high altars on which the sacrifices of truth are placed, so long as they've been carried out in certain ritualistic forms of incantation: introduction, methods, results, conclusions, with special magical symbols in them. One of them is 'p', a strange little symbol that people thought stood for probability but actually stands for publication in some way. So, we head off into that world with its attitudes, and it is difficult, particularly if we meet 'others'—another monkey tribe in the jungle, another set of carers from an entire other culture who act differently. Don't intermingle, and for God's sake don't breed with them. Think of the children. [Laughter.] In fact, since we don't quite understand what they're doing let's burn them, and since we don't know the mechanisms of action of what they do let's burn them good. Do you know, it's only been a hundred and four years since the last witch was burnt (Anna in a Swiss valley)? We should be kind on ourselves; there's a very slowly evolving understanding as a human culture.

Could I have the next slide please? [Slide of the symbol of a locked toilet door—at the bottom of the slide are the words 'Fig diet'.] This is just to suggest reflex activity of the type I've just described. [Laughter.] There's a paradox there, because I think the very parts of us that understand and respond to that symbolism are probably the same parts being moved within the healing encounter. Can I have the next one?

Yes, so here's the ward round at the homoeopathic hospital. [A doctor with a feather head dress dances at the foot of the patient's bed. Patient: 'The headache's still there, Dr Reilly, maybe I could just have an aspirin?' Laughter.] I think there's certainly been a fear of some of the things that I have been discussing and they have been marginalized—much under the term placebo. I'll return to magic later, and try and show you some examples of magic in action. But back to things as usual in our medical world.

Therapeutically, the last few decades, things were going pretty good, making good progress, getting there, except for that damned placebo and its annoying effects. Okay, there are some complications going on, and maybe some side-effects. In Britain last year two and a half thousand people died from bleeding from non-steroidal anti-inflammatory drugs, for example. If that was a new infectious disease can you imagine the multiple-million pounds of research being pumped into it—and the epidemiological scare? Undoubtedly part of the awakening of relooking at things like placebo is trying to find more gentle ways. Can I have the next slide please?

['I'm glad these pills aren't habit forming because I can't do without them.'] Sometimes medicines can be too effective perhaps, and undoubtedly there's too much of them and too many therapies. As you know, by the mid 1980s Valium became the commonest used drug in the world, on the planet, which isn't exactly a glowing example of our sense of balance within our healthcare systems. When I was training I learned that one-third of women around the time of the menopause in the United Kingdom were receiving psychotropic drugs. This is quite intense. What's happening to the therapeutic encounter? We're so very busy aren't we? We're very very busy. Can I have the next slide please? We even equate the business with productivity. [Slide: a person behind a desk responds to the questioner by pointing with a stick to three options on the wall behind: yes/no/I'll talk to you later. Laughter.]

Still, it gives us more time to get down and publish some papers on the placebo response. We have a nurse working in our hospital who's been criticized by her peers for not working enough, and the reason is that she's been tending to sit on the bed of the patients long enough to hold their hands and time to allow them to cry some of those tears—but she's not implementing the nurse practice standard and audit forms efficiently enough. There's may be something fundamentally going wrong in terms of our encounters here. Can I have the next picture please?

[A patient is in a room that is actually a large cage with a hamster exercise wheel in the corner—Is this procedure still experimental doctor? Laughter.] So, having got ourselves in something of a mess, let's go back.

We've become patients and students and carers, so let's go back to being patients again just for a moment, and their instincts and what they've been trying to teach us. A bit like the way dogs eat grass when they're unwell. There's something very ancient, very basic, very instinctive in people who are unwell, who know whether the water's good or bad as I mentioned at the beginning. Some of the stories that I've been hearing over the years from my patients are: 'Well, you know, it is 7-minute appointments and the doctors are so busy', 'I see a different doctor at every visit each time I go to the hospital' 'My name's on the prescription pad before I've sat down on the seat', 'Do you really need to give me drugs doctor; is there not something else?', 'They only wanted to know about a bit of me, and I'm going round various specialists.' Forgive me if I'm being very simple in these things, but it is sometimes these fundamentals that we need to pay more attention to in order to make what we're doing more effective, rather than massive breakthroughs of some type or new fundamental scientific discoveries. Something very simple, something very ordinary and everyday in terms of the quality of our encounter. Can I have the next picture please?

[Commentator to the doctor: 'I am from Which Magazine, we gave this man three fatal diseases and you didn't diagnose one correctly.'] Customer discontent as we all know has led to a massive rise in demand for complementary and alternative medicine—the second biggest growth industry in Europe next to microelectronics, a 3.4 billion dollar industry in Europe. I've been on the interface between the orthodox and alternative world, and I've been well placed to hear the stories. My genuine belief is that the principle thing that's been driving that demand is nothing to do with complementary medicine; it's to do with a heartfelt cry of trying to find some good water, some basic situations that could be summed up, if you like, as good healing encounters, good safe therapy, in a good safe therapeutic environment, from a good safe and wise carer or healer. This is in a way what people were most looking for. Yes it's good to have lots of tools in a tool box, and it's good to have non-toxic, gentle tools first, keeping the stronger medicine as second-line therapy. Yet really at times the issue isn't about the tools or the tool box; the issue is something to do with the encounter. Michaelangelo, if you recall, said that it was just a question of letting the statue that was already there out of the piece of stone. The issue is it's sometimes not the tools that bring the statue out; the tools are the vehicle of the intention in some way, which brings out the situation. I worked for 10 years in the pain relief clinic at the Royal Infirmary in Glasgow in the challenging position of at times seeing the patients after they had failed in the pain relief clinic. In this tough group of patients one of the commonest things to emerge is that these people have not had their story listened to. It's a very simple thing but important thing: they've been to this carer and that carer and they've had 'it' X-rayed, scanned and rubbed and cut and acupuncture needles put in it, yes, and aromatherapy oil rubbed on it, and TENS machines and pain killers, etc., etc. Yet actually to talk about themselves, the events of their life that preceded 'it', and the impact on their self-esteem, to learn something about caring and coping for themselves, getting back on top of the problem, restoring some quality of life, bringing understanding to the change in themselves—this is often not occurring well enough. So, going back now to carers, we need to start to think again. Could I have the next slide?

['My homoeopath and acupuncturist can't help doctor, so in desperation I've come to you.' The circle is beginning to close to some extent. Laughter.] With conferences like this and work that many people have been doing in the last two or three decades, people are beginning to head off and look for other ways. One of those ways that I've been personally involved with is the postgraduate courses in homoeopathy that we've been running in Glasgow. These have become enormously popular. We've trained over 20% of Scotland's general practitioners for example in basic homoeopathy, which is an iceberg that most people don't realize has yet to surface fully in its impact. But what's been most exciting of all I think is to see how easy it is to help the *carers* to transform once more, to be in receipt of some care, to be regiven permission to find again and re-express again some of the basic feelings that took them into medicine—some of the basic empathy and caring attitudes that they hold towards their patients. They're given the okay to begin to look at the whole person, to begin to consider the dynamics of the encounter, to begin to think in terms of subtlety, and to begin to wonder about the possibility of transformation in the encounter. Even sometimes that uncomfortable word 'cure' re-enters the vocabulary having been left many years behind. Let's see the next slide please.

[Slide of a homoeopathic case analysis.] Just to give you a flavour, these are some of the sort of things that might be taken note of with a homoeopathic perspective of someone with inflammatory bowel disease. As well as the usual symptoms and signs of the disease from a Western perspective, the carer is asking about, and more importantly listening to, other elements of disturbance in this person's general well-being and body function, temperature regulation, food cravings, aversions, reactions to the weather, changes in mental content and brain function. Undoubtedly this method has an enormous amount to teach us just about consulting because these encounters are therapeutic in their own right. We need to begin to think of *therapeutic history taking*, the actual act of history taking being an act of therapy—not only a diagnostic act but a therapeutic act, with intention and focus and respect and listening, and wonder, present. This is true often without us actually knowing what 'to do'—taking us back to what I was saying about not understanding life—without us exactly knowing intellectually how these simple elements of compassion and attention bring about transformation and bring out the person's own wisdom and strength in some way.

I mentioned subtlety. It's true that some encounters, like the penicillin and surgery we heard of, are not subtle. That's good, it's great to have those things. We've also heard that even with those very strong interventions the difference between life and death can still rest with the belief of the patient and the circumstances of the encounter. But most of life is even more subtle than that. [Slide.] This is the Atlas Moth, it communicates with its mate through pheromones, airborne hormones, and it's so sensitive that if we put it in human terms it would be like being in London and getting a sniff of your lover in Glasgow. Life is enormously subtle and sensitive, much more subtle and sensitive than modern day medicine. Two or three hundred years from now I think we'll look back on the dark ages of medicine, and on the brutality of much of our current interventions.

Its getting back to the person, to life, to the encounter, to the phenomenon of illness and recovery and healing. Then there are words, and concepts: 'cure, spontaneous remission, regression to the mean, miracle, recovery, catalysed self-healing, placebo, nocebo, transformation, voodoo, electromagnetic fields, prayer, it's χ you see, it's neurolinguistic programming, oh, no, it's psychoneuroimmunology, oh, no, it's shamanism.' I don't know if you get the feel of what I'm trying to say, that something pretty simple, basic, human and core-like is being ripped to shreds in some ways, and cast into territories and into words and into terms, and people are building empires and careers and publications and systems and electronic devices and other things around terms and perceptions of a simple core.

In fact the core phenomena are going on all the time. The things that we're touching on are happening all the time, and not just in the placebo arm of placebo-controlled trials. That's why I'm using such basic words like consultation or encounter. The actual consultation is almost lost within medicine. We must in some way make it conscious.

The anthropological understanding of 'magic' is something to do with shared intention, then a focus; often there are objects around that and rituals are carried out, and then the outcome unfolds. I think I've just described the average consultation. [Laughter.] Whether the object is the prescription pad or the stethoscope, or the temple is a modern hospital with white-coated priests in it, it's happening all the time, and if we're not aware of it happening all the time then we are at risk of unwittingly doing damage all the time. That's why I think it's extremely important for us to study this information and the recent science in some way.

I'd like to show you that magic in action—just to wonder together about these phenomenon. This is something that some of you have seen before (Fig. 7.1) (Reilly & Taylor 1993). These are four individual patients, one graph each, in the context of a double-blind placebo-controlled study (that is, people are receiving dummy medicine or real medicine, and neither the patient nor the carer knows which is which). The charts record the progress of the four patients with asthma over 3 months, with an upward movement

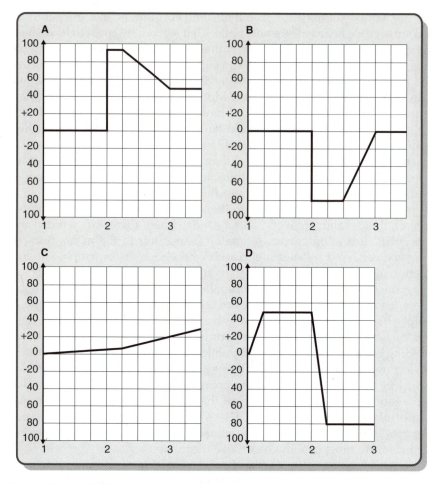

Figure 7.1 The OPIC: overall progress interactive chart. These graphs are redrawn from charts completed interactively by four different patients and their doctor at three visits a month apart during a randomized double-blinded study of a treatment for asthma. The vertical scale is +/– 100%, a rise is an improvement, and the line descends in a deterioration. Point 1 on the horizontal axis marks the first visit when each patient had a *single* blind placebo. Four weeks on at point 2 the patient has been given, randomized and *double* blind, either a second placebo or active medication. At point three a third prescription is given only if required, with those previously randomized to the placebo group again receiving a placebo treatment. The challenge is to determine who got an active medication at the second visit versus who received a second placebo. **A** No response to the first single-blind placebo. Dramatic improvement within hours to the double-blind randomized prescription—ran a marathon! Waned to 50% within about a month. **B** No response to the first single-blind placebo. Dramatic aggravation within hours to the double-blind randomized prescription. 'Worst ever', plus return of old symptoms (rhinitis) and a new symptom of midthoracic back pain. Settled. **C** No response to the first single-blind placebo. A smooth and sustained improvement to the double-blind randomized prescription. **D** Marked improvement with the first single-blind placebo. Dramatic aggravation within hours to the double-blind randomized prescription.

of the line on the graph being an improvement. Now, what most researchers but none of the patients knew was that at time zero the patients received a single-blinded placebo. Then the patients came back a month later and were asked if anything had happened. At this point they received either another placebo or an active medicine. Then they returned again another month later and with the carer they negotiated and drew the graph together as to what happened.

So here's a person (top left graph) who said that he had within hours a dramatic improvement in the asthma to the point that he was able to put his inhalers aside and run the Glasgow marathon! What did he get—active or placebo? Here we have a patient (top right) who had a dreadful dramatic aggravation to the second medicine, so bad that actually he threatened to sue. Another patient (bottom right) had an improvement to the first prescription (placebo) then a deterioration to the second one. Now for the particular therapeutic modality under test I've asked practitioners who received an active prescription at the second point and who received placebo, and how can you tell the difference? The truth is that they all get it wrong, because you can't tell the difference. For if you're speaking about a healing response that is endogenous, and it is being triggered, then the specific therapy will be often using the very same mechanisms as the self-healing systems of the body.

So what people are not understanding about what has been called a placebo response is that this can be a triggering of a true self-healing reaction. Organisms heal, before there were doctors and before there was medicine; organisms heal and they also die and self-destruct. So we're really talking about the true interweaving of the biology and the reactions of the organism with the circumstance and intention and expectation. Three of these four patients received only placebo on both visits. Yet we're seeing here at times even exactly opposite reactions to identical placebos given under identical circumstances by the same caring team. Isn't it remarkable? You know, we don't understand this. Let's be honest with it, we don't really understand how this is transmitted between the players here or how what is transmitted triggers these effects. We know something of how to modify it, amplify it and inhibit it, but we have not been studying this nearly enough. For me the pattern of response of these patients captures something of the excitement and something of the mystery that we're dealing with. Part of the picture is dryly described in the placebo literature as 'the clinicians' expectation of outcome'. At the point the team knew there was a chance of an active medicine at the second visit somehow their expectation has been transmitted. What is it, how is it done? Of course there are many models—whether it's just enthusiasm, tone of voice, whether it could be parapsychological mixed with psychological, we don't really understand. There's a very deep mystery there to be explored.

I'd like in the final part of this chat just to turn to mentioning patients, and the care of individual patients in the context of the search for therapeutic encounters, and say something about my own journey with that. One of the things that's bizarrely ignored in the placebo debate is hypnosis and the hypnotherapeutic literature. It's quite remarkable to me that it's not brought up front and centre stage, even almost as if the concepts are separate. To my perception they're not; to my perception they are mixing and mingling very intimately indeed, and there is a whole literature replete with the question of consciously applied intention and consciously modified intention and what it does in healing. My personal journey was deepened and helped by some years of study of hypnosis and hypnoanalysis, which eventually helped me deepen my capacity to have therapeutic encounters without 'using hypnosis'. I commend to you the thought that it's an illusion that the term placebo and hypnosis are somehow in separate territories or separate places, and that it's an illusion that either of these are somehow separate from the human qualities of encounter and good medicine as I've been trying to emphasize to you.

When I first began to study hypnoanalysis I had some interesting and dramatic times. I remember the case of a girl that I was working with with a more experienced colleague. Every 3 months her hands stopped working; they would curl up in enormous pain and couldn't be touched. She'd had angiograms (X-rays of her blood vessels) and biopsies and had been evaluated for this in many ways other than psychological. She fell into the hands, unfortunately, of a clinical ecologist who in that instance decided that since these paralyses came every 3 months they were probably due to emissions from the local nuclear power station. And so her case deepened. It was very evident that in fact her problems were of a hysterical nature—and there's another word that we need to put aside—because so is a blush: a reaction in the body, not under conscious control, that we didn't want, that we can't stand in front a mirror and order 'go away, you're ruining my life'. We all are subject to such reactions all the time: diarrhoea, sweating, stuttering and so on. And some of it's hived off and medicalized—'this is hysterical paralysis'; then you are off to see the psychiatrists who sometimes don't much know how to handle it anyway, and the situation deepens. So I was doing hypnoanalysis with this girl. I won't tell you of the many adventures that she taught on me during that time, but principally she was taking me towards learning to bridge the gap—the gap between what we call the conscious and the subconscious, which of course again is only our words because it's just us as people and the depths and complexities of us. Anyway, after one of these encounters and catharsis, the crisis, the healing crisis happened. I was pretty sure things were going well when I walked into the ward and she was now paralysed from the neck down! She looked at me smiling, and I smiled back, and I said 'That's fine, that will pass' and so it did, and she was cured. That's now over 10 years ago and she's still well.

As I moved along I began to realize that these types of modifications were not just in what conventional medicine would currently see as 'functional' disorders. I remember one lady on the midway ground between so-called 'organic' and 'functional' illness. She had a weekly positive anti-nuclear factor and an eosinophilia (an increase of certain cells in the blood), the early signs perhaps of a connective tissue disease, and was also suffering from achrocyanosis: shutdown in the blood supply to the hands. She also had sweat that would pour through her clothes, it was so intense, and she had to change her clothes at points throughout the day. She'd been extensively investigated, including whole body CT scans and biopsies of what turned out to be a normal thymus, plus every possible endocrine tumour under the sun had been sought. I'm not saying this disparagingly; I respect and work with the colleague who did this excellent work-up, which I would have required done as well in this instance. But in the end she also healed from a therapeutic encounter that could not so easily be labelled hypnosis—by now I was hovering nervously on the threshold to a place less restricted by these terms. What emerged was a re-evaluation of a near-rape experience at the age of 17, and the frozen terror. When we stepped back and looked afresh I realized the sweat that was pouring off of her body with cold and shaking was the response of a person in terror: a person 'stuck in a blush' if you like, a person stuck in a reaction. Every thought we have, every feeling, floods our body and our system with neurotransmitters and hormones and chemicals, and changes blood flow, and eventually can begin to impact on our tissues and the responses of our tissues.

Then another girl took me a little further. Andrea had been incontinent from the age of 7 and I met her when she was 20. Her bladder would just spontaneously empty. She'd have many good and genuine attempts to help her, but she was holding the appointment card the time that we first met to have her bladder removed in desperation. We had a meeting, which was a human meeting of the type you might begin to sense now that I'm exploring, and she had a spontaneous memory. She suddenly remembered a man running round looking in the toilet windows when she was 7. She was a very strong girl and she was quite convinced that this memory would be the healing of it. But something instinctively was coming to me then that I now begin to understand better, which was a question of timing, and the passage of time in healing work and I said 'It could be, let's see what happens. Come back and see me if you would like.' A year later she came back, still with the same problem, saying that she was still convinced there was something inside but she didn't know what to do. I suggested hypnosis and she said no, she was terrified of hypnosis. She couldn't possibly do that. So I was a bit stuck now. So, as you will when you're challenged, maybe that's the point; you can move a wee bit and I suddenly said: 'Tell me, do you ever daydream?' 'Oh yes, all the time', she said. I said 'Well let's daydream together.' So with eyes open we began to daydream and she wandered through avenues—avenues that neither she nor I yet logically understand I might say. When we finished that daydream she had 24 hours of a sudden and dramatic aggravation and intensification of her problem, and then she was cured—100%. The bladder began to work again. Andrea had had cystometrograms (when you put the dye in the bladder to see if it will contract) and this had been done three times, twice without the general anaesthetic and one with. Even under the general anaesthetic things didn't move.

So we must be dealing with things sometimes here that are as deep into our systems as our innate reflexes of self-protection of life, maybe as intimately linked to this as our breathing and the movement of our hearts. We keep ourselves guarded and defended there whenever we think we must, and so we should, the defence crossing the gap and taking control.

I'd like to tell you about one last patient. By now in my own learning I've reached 1990 and I've abandoned formal procedures such as hypnotherapy and begun to understand that every encounter, like the consultations I discussed with the four patients with asthma earlier, has a state already present, circumstances already set. The person is unwell, they're visiting someone else: 'What will happen?', 'How is this person with me?' 'What am I feeling?', 'What does it mean what they've just said, or not said?' It's happening all the time. Now I am deeply respectful of each encounter. I prepare myself for a few seconds, I try and bring complete attention, complete presence from the moment the person walks in, to be with them, to catch their eye, to touch them if it's appropriate, to ask them how they would like to be called, to sit with them, to listen, to put them at ease. I've discovered that with just those things, combined with basic skills and human skills, remarkable things often happen. Lydia had chronic myeloid leukaemia when she came to see me in mid 1990, and she'd had initial good responses to the hydroxyuria and other chemicals that had been used. But this had stopped working, and she had come along to see me. In my letter back to the referring consultant I emphasized, as I had to her, that although she was seeking homoeopathy at that point, and it could well be added as a complement to the conventional care, it was important not to raise false expectations as there was no evidence that homoeopathy would have a specific action in this disease. Further, I cautioned her against accepting a psychosomatic model as an explanation of her disease, and reminded her that the cause of most disease was still very much unknown.

Then we held a consultation—one in which the room disappeared. What emerged was the death of her husband in 1988, at home, and how she'd nursed him—she was formerly a teacher of French and English and given up her job to nurse him. Her first husband had been alcoholic and she was divorced from him. The problem of the myeloid leukaemia appeared 1 year after the death of her second husband. Telling me this during the consultation, she told me quite logically, quite easily, and she explained that she was fine and was quite happy to die. 'These things happen. I don't mind', she said, 'I'm resigned to it'. I challenged her using something that I had learned through the hypnosis and I now realize is just a natural thing and doesn't need preparation—I said to her without explanation: 'There's a lady sitting behind you and she's 56 and she's got greying hair, and she has chronic myeloid leukaemia and it developed a year after her husband died, and she's just told you that she really doesn't mind dying, she's quite resigned to it. Is there anything you'd like to say to her?' And off she went—explaining to this lady that there was something obviously very wrong with this attitude and that she should now be fighting. This is an example of what I'm trying to hint at, of when one gets beyond the techniques, the words, the systems and returns back to some of the basic human abilities and basic human skills we all have. In speaking to the other woman she began to understand that she had found the metaphor of fighting unacceptable. She had a personality of enormous sensitivity to injustice and cruelty or aggression, and she'd taken on a great deal of self-suppression and non-expression. We talked a little about this. That night back in the hotel, she told me at the next visit, she had had a most profound dream. She was standing in the bath and she was approached by two hands in the air, which reached out and connected to her own and elevated her, actually began to lift her. She said she felt utterly transformed when she awoke, like putting on new clothes. She began to weep in the days that followed, which she'd never managed to do for the death of her husband—wanting him in some ways more and more, as her feelings and her grief emerged.

At the next encounter she told me she was beginning to feel more womanly and she had the reappearance of some sexual feelings. She realized that teaching was no longer satisfying her, and she resolved to make a journey to Australia and undertake a life change. The consultant haematologist noted that she had been transformed and that the disease for now seemed to have normalized. She said 'I'm dreaming in primary colours for the first time in years'. When she returned from Australia she told me a story, but by now there is an awkwardness in me as I realize she's more alive than I am. It's very interesting (a word I use to cover discomfort). She comes back to tell me about the freedom that's developed in her life, and the experiences that she's having. She's radiating. She's teaching me basically and I'm almost shy now of the situation, watching and learning from her. She went into the desert in Australia with an Aboriginal guide, who told her she would have an animal guide, and lo and behold a small bird appeared and stayed with her for 2 days, flying around her and following her through the desert. Radiant and full of life and quite transformed she lived another 3 years. At the end she wrote to me releasing me from my care for her in a way that left me speechless.

The last image I'd like to leave with you is this slide of a hand in a candle flame. It is Emaho's hand—a contemporary shaman. I've watched this now maybe 12 times and studied it on a video that I made. Emaho prepares, then places his hands directly in the candle flame for many minutes. This is part of his preparation for the healing encounters he then has with people. At first my mind clicked in and offered all sorts of explanations— altered states, you know, theta waves, hypnosis, this is this, this is that, and then I began to soften a wee bit after seeing it a few times, to begin to realize that such mechanisms might control the pain—but they would not stop fire burning tissue. I don't know what this is and I'd like to stop now on the idea that there are perhaps quite profound unknown depths still to be explored in healing work. Thank you very much. [Applause]

QUESTIONS FROM FLOOR

The questioner asks how the process of therapeutic consulting could be taught. Until a year ago I felt unable to allow a video camera or anyone else into the consultation. Because of the loss of sanctity and privacy. But it has become obvious to me that I have a responsibility to try to teach. So I have asked my senior house officers to sit in with me for the last year, and try taking notes and they have begun to teach me how I might teach what I am doing. Their insights help me see some of the components and processes involved. And in fact in the workshop that I'm doing I have the first two pages of a little draft from the senior house officers' reflection on what I do. But I think that it can be taught; much of it is by seeing it and feeling it, and realizing the simplicity of it; the absolute naturalness of it. And in a sense receiving permission to become yourself, to become more yourself, to be more relaxed and more present in the situation.

The questioner suggests that the placebo idea is actually a two-way thing, and that the possibility of deceit is something to be considered. Yes, that's why I think we should be careful about reviving the term placebo and linking it with all the healing potential that lives in the consultation and the therapeutic relationship. Better that we should begin to talk about healing responses and self-healing responses and self-destructive responses, and legitimize their study. As patients and as carers we need to understand how to enhance the healing process, and what inhibits it. And one thing that inhibits it is deceit. And it is too easy for conventional medical audiences sometimes to misunderstand and to think I want to encourage the use of placebos—which is the exact opposite of what I'm trying to say. Because I don't believe that as a carer or as a patient you should be involved in a healing encounter unless you feel safe and comfortable, and authentic and genuinely believe in what you are doing.

Which is where our science and our training and our discipline are so important. We should bring ourselves to a point of complete honesty in the encounter. We have to hunt down self-illusion and woolly thinking. We have to resist the idea that rigour and training don't matter and 'so let's just all get together and do healing work'.

The questioner has spoken about the man I mentioned in casualty who received saline, saying he was deceived but it worked, so does it really matter? For me, yes, it matters deeply. Because that man's problem was not resolved by any means. His understanding wasn't deepened, in fact his problem was probably deepened, his relationship with his carers was disturbed, and I wouldn't feel good about the likely next event, when that man gets unwell the next time around. I don't think I would have injected saline into anyone. No, I think I would have been with him and done whatever came naturally under the circumstances, to help him understand, to bring his anxiety down, to do what needs to be done.

The question is about the lady with the bladder difficulty and whether the inherent conflicts were symbolized into the dreams and whether that shed some light. Yes and no. I think we are at the beginning of learning the language of the inner world. We enter it for many hours every night, and we think of it as almost a foreign territory, as if it had nothing to do with us. We say 'It wasn't me, it was my subconscious' … or … 'I don't know why I did that, it just came out'. And as a culture we are living in a moment where that gap is quite enormous. I imagine that before there was consciousness, even in evolutionary terms, much of our interaction with the environment was of course through our senses, through vision and through smell and through touch and through image, and through the recalling of those images. And that's why in my own work I find the most powerful tool perhaps is metaphor, it's therapeutic metaphor, and accepting that metaphor and myth are the same as dreams, and are accessible to us all the time. They touch us and activate us. So a story told at the right moment can be very, very healing.

One that touched me and that I like to tell my patients is: 'Did you hear about the Chinese tomb that was discovered about 19 years ago? They found some seeds in the tomb and they were approximately two and half thousand years old, these seeds, and they planted them and they actually germinated, and they grew into a magnolia tree. And 18 months ago I saw this story again in the media because the tree had flowered, after all that wait.' And I think sometimes a story like this told during an effective encounter, when something is actually present in the atmosphere, can help unlock the healing that's stuck in people. It's like the flow of water, if things are dammed back you maybe remove one brick and the water begins to trickle and then it begins to flow. And you don't need to run ahead of it saying turn left, turn right, do this, hey watch that boulder; there's something about life and the way it moves and there's something about the way healing moves: that it knows what to do, that you be given permission and touch it.

So, here was this girl with me, trusting me, present with me, entering the safety of the daydream with me, accepting the gentle prompts that we might drift backwards and see what would emerge. And out came some story related to her sister, and she and her sister are running in some way, and there's danger around, and she's falling and stumbling and has to pick her sister up and keep running. The emotion is rising and one can see the physical changes in the body occurring at that time. But there's no wonderful logical resolution. Perhaps just being there saying that's okay and it's all right, and then coming out of the daydream and the thing is resolved. And one of the things I've had to learn is that thank goodness we don't need to tell the water how to flow.

You were making a point about the intellectualization of the process: the need to find a firm interpretation. I think we need to let go of that a bit because even though the dreams generated are helpful and can often be understood, sometimes they are not. And that can still be all right.

The questioner asks about the hand in the candle, and the rose also not burning. He asks whether this is a metaphor and whether I have used such metaphors. I would like to try and address both the questions you asked in terms of a metaphor and not as a metaphor. As a metaphor first of all: yes, the courage that's in us to deal with say the death that approaches or the cancer that's not curable, or the pain that won't go away, to water the seeds of hope, to bring back something of an original feeling of connectedness to life and to ourselves, and some of the okayness within that, then I think yes, sometimes stories that tell of light and of strength and of courage and of endurance are good. They can help reawaken our strength.

I think, at this stage for me, the challenge is in seeing that image also as a reality. Because at first I couldn't engage with the reality. I had to deal with it as metaphor and find an explanation. And now I can't allow that in myself any more. And I have been present in what this man, Emaho, calls a fire dance: not walking on hot coals, but him and these candles, and him placing his hands in the candle flame and then taking people one at a time to dance for a few seconds. And I think what he's trying to teach us is that we are alive, actually are alive: that the fire in us is good and that it can be awakened. But I do not have any intellectual understanding whatsoever of this process. I have had some experiential understanding of it with him, some quite profound experiences with it. And that is why I believe I am now prepared to open up to the fact that there is more going on here than just psychological healing. There's something else, there's something about life and its power and its healing potential. And that, for me, is getting on to what feels like pretty scary ground.

The next questioner says he thinks I have suggested that we are all already in a trance, and that therefore formal trance induction is unnecessary. I would agree with that, but I would abandon the term 'trance' altogether. I would actually say that we are alive all the time; that we are responding and being touched and moved and moving the world around us, and relating to the people and circumstances around us, but that we do not realize it enough. We are not present in it enough. So for instance as we walk past and subliminally catch that look in the eye of the doctor or the nurse, something significant is happening and something is moving all the time. Or if you return home and walk back into your house and the atmosphere isn't good. You know it. Okay. And maybe it's the way your wife is clonking the dishes in the dishwasher, and you haven't gone in the room yet and you know it. Okay. I think that's what I'm trying to say, that if we could embrace it and bring it into our healing world in an ordinary way, then I think we'd get much better results.

The next questioner thinks I was poking fun a wee bit at the scientific method. Perhaps I do! And that the information I am gathering could be made accessible to scientific enquiry. Yes, of course, and I would definitely consider myself a scientist but also an artist too. So I check out what I am doing from different directions. I want evidence, I don't just want ideas. We all need to be aware that our capacity for wisdom is matched by that for self-delusion. Science is one of the ways to understand what we work with, and we have to call on it when appropriate.

The questioner observed there is some evidence that you can explain placebo to the client and then use it effectively. Yes, but I wouldn't use the word placebo as a way of explaining the process. I might speak of life, of healing, of learning to cope again, of getting back on your feet. I might tell stories about that from other people and tell of examples where transformation happened. I might talk about people realizing what had happened and how they had fallen and how they might brush the mud off and start walking again, and find resources within themselves. I might speak of the long time that could take and some of the energies that can sustain one when you keep falling down again with your face in the mud. But I don't use the term placebo at any point. The only time I use the term placebo these days is as a hook or anchor point in the beginning of communication, particularly with my orthodox medical colleagues. Because it's a current word and it's a good starting point. Of course, intention is like a laser that moves out in front of us: the star that guides us. And if you expect trivia you get trivia. Intention: I decide to move my arm, my arm moves. I decide that even though in my head is an image of the person who hurt me and that I want to kick to death, I move somehow else. So instead I become a doctor and learn to meet people and sit with them and to believe that it can bring benefits. Yes, so I think loving, caring, humanness, are qualities that we intend. There is a quote from Emaho; he said: 'the power of the Sun is like a candle flame compared to the power of kindness'.

REFERENCES

Blackwell B, Bloomfield S S, Buncher C R 1972 Demonstration to medical students of placebo responses and non-drug factors. Lancet 13:1–11
Reilly D T, Taylor M A 1993 The Overall Progress Interactive Chart. In: Developing integrated medicine. Report of the RCCM Fellowship in Complementary Medicine. University of Glasgow 1987–90. Complementary Therapies in Medicine 1(suppl 1):1–50

7

Psychoanalysis, complementary medicine and the placebo

Robert Withers

Editor's note

Bob Withers is a rare combination: a trained Jungian analyst who is also an acupuncturist and a homoeopath. His MPhil research explored the psychology of homoeopathy and as an analyst he is committed to the idea that the unconscious is all around and constantly at work. His concern in this chapter is with communication at a deeper level: of a kind that almost always evades our attention. It has been said that the existence of placebo effects demonstrates that nothing goes into the mouth without going through the imagination too. Bob might well respond that nothing enters consciousness without also making unfelt waves beneath our everyday awareness. This idea should certainly make us more curious about the role of the imagination in healthcare, and particularly the impact of complementary therapy with its rich images and mysterious intentions. Bob invites us to consider two examples: one explores the imaginal power of acupuncture and its needles; the other looks at some interesting undercurrents in a homoeopathic case. Both are disciplines whose underlying theories and approach to history taking strikingly blur the distinction between mind and body. Bob looks at the implications of this important common feature, then shifts his perspective to show how consultations often reflect unacknowledged or unspoken emotional difficulties; and most significantly the life issues that practitioner and client share. He comes to the conclusion that the most effective consultations occur when the patient feels the clinician's intervention has somehow made these unspeakable elements safe. Bob suggests that in these and other ways the unfolding therapeutic relationship can unfreeze stagnant self-healing processes, and perhaps even more interestingly that this containment may be conveyed not only through language (the psychotherapist's way) but also by what is enacted in the complementary therapy consultation and treatment.

INTRODUCTION

It is generally acknowledged that the placebo effect accounts for a large part of the effectiveness of any medical intervention. Yet surprisingly little has been written on its operation from a psychoanalytic point of view. Arguably this is because of reluctance among analysts to trespass into the domain of the body. This has traditionally become the territory of hard science ever since Descartes' liberation of scientific knowledge from religion in the seventeenth century. In this deal modern men and women appear to have gained the world but lost their souls! Psychoanalysis may seem to some people an odd vehicle with which to attempt a postmodern re-ensoulment of medicine. But I would argue that its reliance on intro-spection makes it ideally placed to accomplish this task. It is just this introspective element that the cartesian paradigm effectively ruled out of modern medicine. Michael Balint (1957) attempted to pioneer its reintro-duction to orthodox medicine. In this chapter I hope to extend his work by showing how an analytic understanding of complementary medicine can help illuminate the operation of the placebo effect. In order to do this, I will begin by telling a story.

ACUPUNCTURE AND THE PLACEBO

Some 15 years ago, when I was a recently qualified acupuncturist, a man walked into my consulting room suffering from acute rheumatoid arthritis. He was a small man in his late twenties, with a pronounced fear of needles. His symptoms were severe enough to keep him off work and he had tried conventional treatment without any lasting success. He had turned to acupuncture in desperation but was too frightened in the first session to allow me to insert any needles. Instead we talked about the origins of his fear, in the hope that if we could understand it he might be able to overcome it enough to let me treat him in the next session.

Mr X as I shall call him was one of those people who have an intuitive grasp of their own psychology without ever having been in therapy, and with very little prompting from me he went on to describe his relationship as a boy with his much-loved grandmother. She was a large and friendly woman, and he was in the habit, of a morning, of climbing into her bed and romping about before she got up. He recalled with obvious emotion a particular incident as a 6-year-old child. On the morning in question, he climbed into her bed as usual, but noticing she was very still he began tugging at her to wake her up. Eventually he succeeded in rolling her over, but to his horror she fell out of bed, pinning him to the floor underneath her. Trapped and panicking, his cries eventually alerted the other adults, who came and removed her dead body from on top of him. She had died in the night, and he dated his fear of being trapped and helpless, and hence his fear of acupuncture, to this incident.

Following this account, Mr X gradually became able to tolerate my needles, and I began treating him according to the principles of Traditional Chinese Medicine. He responded well, and within a few treatments was able to return to work and gradually reduce the frequency of his sessions.

Things progressed in a satisfactory if unspectacular manner until one day when he missed an appointment. It so happened at this time that I was having trouble with people cancelling appointments in what I considered a casual manner, and having recently started psychotherapy myself, where missed sessions are charged for, I decided to tackle him about it when he turned up for his next session. In order to do this I chose the time when he was lying on the couch, with the needles in, as this is a fallow time not taken up with what I considered the more important business of information gathering and diagnosis. He told me that on the day in question he had set out as usual for his appointment, only to find that British Rail had changed their timetable. He said he understood that I had lost my income for that session, but did not feel inclined to pay the fee himself, since the change in timetable was not his fault. I commented that it was not my fault either. In the end, we settled on a compromise whereby he paid half the fee and, apparently satisfied, he walked out.

I was horrified when he hobbled in wracked with pain for his next session. The redness and swelling had returned to his joints, and he was off work again, in as bad a state as when I had first seen him. My first thought was to check my treatment notes, but there was nothing unusual about the points I had used. Next I asked whether he had done anything different himself since we had last met, but he said he hadn't. Puzzled and disappointed, I could see no option but to continue with the treatment as usual, which I did.

When the session ended he thanked me for my help, but said that he didn't want to spend any more money on a treatment that had stopped working. As he left he turned to me one last time, and asked whether I thought the mind could have an effect on the body. I said I was sure it could, but asked him what he meant. In time now outside the official session, he proceeded to tell me with great vehemence how I had made him feel in the previous session. I had known about his fear of being trapped so he found it incredible that I had chosen his time on the couch to confront him about the money. He had felt pinned down by me and my needles, and unable to express his anger about being charged anything for a session he had missed through no fault of his own. He attributed the return of his symptoms directly to this experience and went on in this vein until exactly half a session's worth of time had passed. Then he turned and left, leaving me feeling crushed.

Reflection

The first point I realized in reflecting about this case was the importance of the therapeutic relationship to the outcome of treatment. And if an interaction like that described above could have such a profound negative effect then conceivably the same could be true of the positive influence of a different kind of interaction. If this were the case, it would seem plausible that factors in the therapeutic relationship could form the basis of much of what passes for the placebo effect.

A second point is that understanding the basis of this patient's negative therapeutic reaction (or nocebo effect) depended on taking his introspection seriously. It would have been all too easy to overlook this. An objective account of this case would not have considered his feelings of anger. And yet, as I hope to show later, once those feelings are noticed and taken seriously a plausible account of their connection to symptom aggravation can be given. In a similar way the influence of the therapeutic relationship on the outcome can be untangled only if the practitioner's thoughts, feelings and actions are also noticed and taken seriously. This takes the practitioner out of the place of objective observer and into the realm of the interactive participant.

A third point is that what is true here of acupuncture seems likely to be true of many, if not all, forms of medical intervention. Naturally the precise means of operation of placebo and nocebo effects will vary from therapy to therapy, and even within the same therapy, as the symptoms differ and the dynamics of the interaction change. But I would argue that a close consideration of those dynamics can illuminate the operation of both placebo and nocebo effects within a wide variety of therapies. And I hope to illustrate this later on by considering the placebo effect in the treatment of a homoeopathic patient.

Fourthly, it should be noted that the resolution of a nocebo effect is as likely to enhance a treatment as the evocation of the placebo effect itself. Thus placebo and nocebo effects are inextricably linked. This point is well illustrated by Mr X himself. Six months after the above session, he referred a work colleague to me, who had obviously been impressed by the effects of my treatment. Mr X, the latter said, considered himself cured! Some 12 years after this Mr X himself came back for a different problem and wondered somewhat sheepishly if I remembered him. I assured him that I did, and in response to my enquiries he told me that he had been more or less symptom free since his last visit. Presumably something about that final interaction had reversed the nocebo effect of the previous session. But what exactly had caused the nocebo effect in the first place and what had happened in the final session to enhance its resolution? In order to attempt to answer these questions it will be useful first to make a brief philosophical digression and then to introduce a few key psychoanalytic concepts.

Mind–body link

The specific question I wish to consider is how could psychological factors have precipitated the return of Mr X's physical symptoms—and especially the palpable swelling and redness of his joints? Analysts are inclined to gloss over such awkward questions with an appeal to concepts like the defence of somatization. But such notions tend to beg the question of how the jump from mind to body occurs in the first place.

The most plausible account I know of this mind–body leap in rheumatoid arthritis (RA) sufferers occurs in Herbert Weiner's book psychobiology and human disease (1977). He draws on the earlier studies of Franz Alexander (1950), himself a student of Freud's. Weiner postulates that RA sufferers are genetically predisposed to produce an inflammatory reaction to breakdown products of their own bodies accumulating in their joints (hence the rheumatoid factors in their blood). These breakdown products, he argues, are increased in amount if the muscles around a joint are tense, the ensuing wear and tear on the joint becoming correspondingly greater. One can imagine my patient tensing his muscles in a state of powerless rage as I confronted him about the fees for the missing session. He may have carried this rage and tension around with him until he was able to discharge it by telling me how he felt and by 'reclaiming' the missing half-session in his final appointment. In the intervening time the build-up of breakdown products and the inflammatory reaction to them may have been so great that it resulted in the palpable changes I observed.

Of course, this account is far from being either complete or a generic description of the mind–body link in the placebo effect. But it seems plausible, and it is likely that similar mechanisms involving different pathways exist in other cases as well. The effect of psychological factors on endorphins, gastric secretions, blood pressure and the immune system is well documented (e.g. Watkins 1997) and their influence on sexuality, breathing, posture and the voluntary muscles, as well as general behaviour, cannot be doubted. All these systems could eventually influence a wide variety of physical symptoms, and so psychological factors affecting them could easily contribute to placebo and nocebo effects.

Assuming some such account is eventually possible in most placebo incidents, the jump from mind to body that at first appeared so surprising resolves itself into a philosophical problem: how is it that any mental phenomenon can affect any physical one? To use Descartes' terminology: how can thinking unextended substance (mind) affect unthinking extended substance (body)? Of course our minds affect our bodies every time we perform a voluntary action. So there is no practical problem here. But, following Wittgenstein (1958), the problem in conceiving of such interactions becomes one of discourse or, as he called it, 'language games'. When medicine adopted the discourse of objective science, it generally excluded the discourse of feelings and introspection. The two belonged to different language games. Thus for some time it became nonsensical for scientific medicine even to ask how feelings might affect physical symptoms.

Linked into this philosophical problem is one of distribution of power. According to Foucault (1970) medical power depends upon privileging the discourse of objective measurable observation (the mathesis), over other discourses such as that of introspection. Its reintroduction is then essentially subversive of that power. But I believe that it is at least in part this threat that lies behind the general exclusion of the discourse of introspection and psychoanalysis from conventional Western medicine. However, as patients and practitioners alike demand that their therapies become more holistic, that exclusion becomes increasingly untenable. Its reintroduction may result in the loss of the kind of certainty that characterizes much of Western medicine. But its continued exclusion arguably results in a greater loss (medical soul loss).

It will be necessary next to introduce five key analytic concepts to the proceedings.

Analytic concepts

Psychoanalytic terminology evolved within the context of a culturally specific set of assumptions about the nature of the self and the world. Postmodern critiques implicitly challenge those assumptions, and in so doing reveal Western individualism (and the cartesian dualism on which it is based) as just one possible way among many of experiencing the world and ourselves. Paradoxically, contemporary psychoanalysis with its emphasis on the unconscious and upon language (see e.g. Lacan 1949) is instrumental in deconstructing the very world view upon which it is predicated. Nevertheless in order to give a simple outline of the five basic analytic concepts below it is necessary to refer implicitly to that world view.

1. Projection

When people are unable to acknowledge consciously certain qualities or experiences as properly belonging to themselves, they may experience them as coming from outside. That is, they may attribute them rightly or wrongly to other people (or things) via projection.

2. Transference

The term 'transference' has come to be used in contemporary analysis to cover all the patient's thoughts and feelings about the therapist (see, for example, Bateman & Holmes 1995). This is, however, a broader definition than that originally put forward by Freud (1914). He saw the transference, more narrowly, as a repetition in the present of unconscious elements of a past relationship. An example of transference of this kind occurs in the above case. Mr X came into treatment with a fear of needles, which he himself attributed to his past experience with his grandmother. This was repeated in the present in relation to me via projection. He feared I would be like his dead granny and pin him down with my needles. Once this negative transference became conscious and was put into words (symbolized) his anxiety was reduced and he was able to allow me to use needles.

The situation becomes at once more complex and more interesting, however, if the memory of his grandmother evokes something of the present as well as the past. She could for instance stand for a feared crushing, dead part of himself that threatens at times to overwhelm his more vulnerable self either directly or via projection on to others. Considerations such as this have led contemporary analysts to extend their use of the term transference to cover all of the patient's thoughts and feelings about the therapist. According to this view past and present, perception and projection, are inextricably linked and the transference is therefore likely to contain all these elements.

3. Countertransference

Just as the term transference has undergone evolution, so too has the term 'countertransference'. It originally referred to the therapist's unconsciously determined neurotic reaction to the patient, and was regarded as detrimental to treatment. Later it came to signify all the therapist's thoughts and feelings about the patient and its positive aspects were recognized (Bateman & Holmes 1995). Thus my failure to appreciate Mr X's sensitivity to feeling trapped as I interrogated him about money almost certainly had neurotic elements. Like him I had a well-loved grandmother who died when I was 6, and my own unresolved feelings about this could have created a blind spot, which somehow contributed to my insensitivity. In addition, like many practitioners in private practice, I probably felt guilty about asking my patients for money at all, let alone money for missed sessions. An unconscious overcompensation for this could easily have contributed to my insensitivity. No doubt I also had (and have!) sadistic elements in my personality, which I was perhaps unconsciously acting out. These then are all examples of countertransference in its original sense.

But, in addition to all my own neurosis, it seems likely that I actually behaved like a crushing dead granny because he projected that part of himself on to me. If he hadn't already been projecting it on to me, he would probably have felt safe enough to tell me how I was making him feel with my insensitive questioning, and our interaction could have changed. In that sense then my countertransference was reactive as well as neurotic.

4. Projective identification

When therapists end up feeling or behaving in the same way as patients unconsciously expect or fear they will, they could be said to have identified with patients' projections. The analytic term for this is 'projective identification'. Since patients often split off and project unacceptable parts of themselves on to others (in this case a crushing dead part), it follows that therapists may be able to learn something about their patient's most problematic areas by reflecting on their own behaviour, thoughts or feelings—that is, by introspecting. Naturally a therapist working in this way needs some experience in attempting to separate neurotic from reactive elements in the countertransference, otherwise they may simply end up blaming the patient for their own difficulties—or vice versa. To assist in this task, most of us would find personal therapy and individual supervision helpful.

Another example of projective identification occurred in the final session when I ended up feeling crushed by him as he presumably had by me in the previous session. Of course the anxiety associated with this experience probably stirred up feelings that originated with the incident as a boy when his grandmother's dead body crushed him.

5. Containment

If projective identification has a purpose apart from the evacuation of unpleasant experiences or feelings into someone else, it is to seek help from them in managing those feelings. Thus Mr X's unconscious hope in crushing me in the final session may have been to enlist my help in his ongoing attempt to transform the unbearable anxiety associated with his grandmother's death and his own experience of being crushed by her into a form that he could contain himself. Bion (1962) likens this to a process of detoxification. Once people are able to contain their detoxified feelings in this way, they can represent them symbolically in language, thought or dream, without being overwhelmed by anxiety. This capacity to contain them may need to be encountered in the other before it can be internalized and finally made the subject's own. The process of internalizing detoxified projections like this has been termed 'reintrojection'.

An example of a failure to contain and detoxify projections occurred in the penultimate session when I acted like the patient's crushing granny without realizing it. The result of this was an escalation rather than containment of his anxiety.

Although the above glossary of terms is based upon the individualistic notion of one person projecting the contents of his unconscious into another separate person, it is worth noting that it also implicitly undermines that individualism. In projection I look out and encounter the self, whereas in projective identification I look in and encounter the other.

Factors within the therapeutic relationship

Having established the use of the salient analytic terms (and also touched on some other) I can now turn to a consideration of the influence of the therapeutic relationship on the outcome of treatment in the case of Mr X. The three sessions with most relevance here are the first and last two sessions.

The first session

The relevant point relating to the first session seems to be that I represented the crushing dead granny in the transference. By adapting my normal procedure, mastering my impatience and not inserting needles I unconsciously began the task of containing and detoxifying this projection. That is I did not behave in the insensitive way he feared or expected. This contributed to the resolution of Mr X's negative transference, helped him to tell me about his experience with his grandmother and enabled him to enter treatment.

For his part, the decisive factor was his articulation of the story about his grandmother, which helped him contain his anxiety in language—that is, represent his experience symbolically. It was now well enough bound not to stand in the way of effective treatment for a while at least.

The penultimate session

If I succeeded in containing and detoxifying his projections in the first session, in the penultimate session I spectacularly failed to do so. In contrast, I actually behaved like the feared dead grandmother. My insensitive behaviour resulted in the return of his projections in an unmodified form, and the escalation of his anxiety. This eventually led to an exacerbation of his symptoms and the breakdown of the therapeutic relationship.

The final session

Many of the issues arising in the final session have been touched on already but, at the risk of repeating myself, I will now try briefly to draw them together.

The first point to note is that the return of Mr X's symptoms can be regarded as an expression of the negative transference, which had been triggered in the previous session when I behaved like his crushing dead grandmother. When he became able to symbolize those feelings by telling me how I had made him feel, this removed the need to express them through muscular tension with the ensuing effects. The improvements of the preceding sessions could then reinstate themselves.

He also seems to have needed a means of acting out his feelings. He did this by offering me an exchange. He could give me some very interesting information (while also telling me off) in return for me making up the extra time I had made him pay for in the previous session. He could then leave with his honour intact and myself suitably crushed but enlightened.

It was probably this vulnerable terrified feeling of being crushed that he found hardest to bear. Pushing it into me via projective identification like this is therefore likely to have given him some instant relief. But it is also possible that seeing me contain it to a certain extent helped him manage it better for himself in the long run. Putting this in analytic terms, we might say that perhaps my capacity to survive being crushed by him without retaliating enabled him to somehow reintroject something of that capacity for himself.

From a strictly psychoanalytic point of view this exchange could be looked on as a failure. Technically I broke a boundary by staying to listen to him into my lunch hour. And he broke off treatment before a range of important unconscious material could be made conscious. On the other hand a number of therapeutic interactions appear to have occurred without needing to be made conscious, and Mr X got what he came for in terms of symptom relief. I also gained some invaluable experience early on in my practice. So perhaps within the parameters of an acupuncture treatment it could be viewed as a success even if the ending was rather traumatic! It also seems likely that he continued to reflect on his experience with me, and in this sense his therapeutic work continued after the end of our sessions (as of course did mine).

Factors outside the therapeutic relationship

I hope that the above account shows how the language of psychoanalysis can help illuminate factors within the therapeutic relationship that are of relevance to understanding the placebo effect. I will move on shortly to consider the application of the same concepts to a homoeopathic case.

Before doing so, however, I wish to acknowledge that there are many non-specific factors outside the therapeutic relationship with a potential bearing on outcome and hence the placebo effect. Some of these, such as the quality of the patient's other relationships, could also be talked about in analytic terms. But unfortunately a full discussion of them lies outside the parameters of the present chapter.

HOMOEOPATHY AND THE PLACEBO

In this section I will attempt to show how the analytic concepts outlined above can be of use in articulating some of the placebo factors at work in a specific fairly ordinary homoeopathic case. I will go on to consider whether they can help with a more general elucidation of placebo factors within homoeopathy.

A young mother consulted me some 10 years ago for homoeopathic treatment of multiple symptoms. These included lower- and upper-back pain, a tendency to starve and binge on food, digestive problems and lack of interest in sex. She had a history, amongst other things, of migraine and dragging uterine pains. She had recently arrived in this country with her husband and two young boys, and had been treated homoeopathically for slightly different symptoms with mixed results in her country of origin. Her husband, a carpenter, was finding it difficult to get work here. She herself was training in one of the caring professions. There were money worries. In addition, although she described her older son as 'good', her younger one was having problems at school, and at times she found his behaviour difficult and got irritated with him.

Mrs A as I shall call her seemed a typical Sepia case, and so I prescribed Sepia 200. After a short initial aggravation, she gradually improved over a course of monthly consultations. The Sepia 200 was too dilute to contain a single molecule of the cuttle fish ink from which it originated. Homoeopathic sceptics would therefore argue that her improvement must have been entirely due to placebo factors. On the other hand most convinced homoeopaths would consider that the Sepia worked physically in some way beyond the current understanding of science. Whatever the truth about the remedy, were there any factors in the therapeutic relationship that might have contributed to her improvement? If so what were they?

The role of the relationship

Countertransference

At the time of treating Mrs A I did not pay particular attention to my countertransference feelings towards her. All these years later though I am aware of a dynamic I didn't allow myself to dwell upon too closely at the time. Mrs A had been telling me about her financial problems. I had then examined her back. While she was getting off my examination couch, her short skirt rode up her thighs revealing two fairly large holes high up the inside leg of her tights. The fact that I can recall this image so vividly now indicates that there was certainly an erotic element in my countertransference. But I can also recall having some protective feelings towards her— something along the lines of 'If you were my wife I'd make sure you didn't have to wear such tattered underwear'.

Transference

With the benefit of hindsight I can see that my erotic feelings were probably reciprocated, at least unconsciously, since Mrs A turned her bottom towards me and lingered for a fraction of a second before pulling her skirt down after getting off the couch.

Erotic playback

All this happened without being remarked on at the time, and probably remained largely unconscious. But it brings to mind the work of Andrew Samuels (1993) and other analysts on erotic playback. According to Samuels, a young girl is helped to grow into a sexually viable woman if her father is able to communicate that he finds her sexually attractive, while maintaining clear sexual boundaries for her. Sometimes fathers disrupt their daughter's sexual development by breaking the incest taboo and the damage can be devastating. But it is probably even more common for them to inflict the opposite kind of damage by acting too coldly. Such an attitude conveys the unconscious message that sexuality is so dangerous that it must be vigorously defended against. And the girl may grow into a woman who feels she has to suppress her own sexual feelings. Another way of putting this is to say that the father's difficulty in containing his sexual feelings towards his daughter may lead to her having difficulties in containing and thus consciously enjoying hers later in life. Her sexual feelings may then come to be experienced as toxic to her psyche, especially if anxiety is already high for other reasons, such as stressful life circumstances.

Much of this seems likely to have applied to Mrs A, contributing to the loss of sexual feelings towards her husband. Those feelings seem to have resurfaced in relation to me when I examined her back, however. And perhaps the fact that I neither rejected nor took advantage of them helped her to internalize the containment she needed to take them back into the relationship with him. This could help account for the improvement in their relationship, and in turn could have had a knock-on effect on her other symptoms, most obviously the lower-back pain.

Before moving on from the theme of the transference and countertransference, it seems worth commenting on the fact that Mrs A's story also elicited feelings of care and sympathy in me. She presented herself like an orphan adrift in a strange world, and I responded by feeling protective towards her. It seems likely that she picked up on this through little clues. For instance as I thanked her for my fee I found myself asking 'are you sure that's all right?' in a way that showed my concern without denying my own need to eat. Events such as this may have helped her to contain her own feelings of dependency at a time when she generally felt she had to suppress her needs in order to go on looking after the many others in her care. Each time she took one of her remedies at home she may have been reminded of this experience. This in turn could have helped relieve some of her eating and digestive disorders since eating feels dangerous to people who are afraid of their own dependency needs (Eichenbaum & Orbach 1985), and digestion can easily become upset by irregular eating patterns and strong emotions.

Taking the remedy could also have helped improve her relationship with her son since she is likely to have felt less resentful towards him and his needs now that some of her own were beginning to feel more contained. I also believe however that there were other ways in which the homoeopathic consultation and remedy may have contributed to placebo factors in her recovery.

The consultation

We saw above how notions derived from psychoanalysis such as transference, countertransference and containment could be used to help clarify placebo events in both an acupuncture and a homoeopathic case. It is my contention that such events are far from rare, occurring regularly in many forms of medical treatment. As mentioned previously the GP and analyst Michael Balint (1957) attempted to pioneer an analytic exploration of them within orthodox medicine. The adoption of this approach was hampered, however, by the lack of time available for the average GP consultation, coupled with a general medical preoccupation with objective rather than subjective information gathering (Pietroni 1989).

The situation is very different in complementary medicine where not only is more time available, but also the practitioner is interested in all the patient's symptoms including, and sometimes especially, the subjective ones. This is because homoeopathic remedies, like acupuncture points and other holistic treatments, are usually chosen on the basis of a combination of subjective and objective symptoms. It is true that, unlike the analytical psychotherapist, the complementary practitioner is generally not trained to make conscious use of transference/countertransference events such as those outlined above. But this does not mean that they do not occur. Indeed many years' experience first as a complementary therapist and then as an analytical psychotherapist has taught me that they are actually more likely to occur in the former than in the latter context.

It is worth noting here that Freud (1893) first observed the existence of the transference when Anna O. fell in love with his colleague Joseph Breuer who was treating her with a hypnotherapeutic technique involving massage. It seems likely that it was the combination of physical with psychological contact that allowed the transference to emerge with such force (a force incidentally that Breuer reciprocated to the extent that it almost destroyed his marriage).

So it could well be that the analytic insistence on abstinence from touch was developed to help diminish the intensity of such disturbing events. If this is the case it would mean that often holistic practitioners are working in the midst of powerful forces they generally have no training even to recognize let alone work therapeutically with. This does not mean effective therapeutic work cannot be done. It often is. But it seems likely that the potential therapeutic benefits of working consciously with the transference and countertransference are radically diminished whereas the potential for causing harm is correspondingly increased. In particular there is a real danger of sexual misconduct that is damaging to both patient and practitioner. This is far too common even with fully trained counsellors and psychotherapists where no touch is involved. When it is, and the training to deal with and understand it is even less, the risks may seem unacceptably high. It is at such times that the temptation to ignore the psyche or the body, or retreat behind a desk wearing a white coat and gloves, can become overpowering! We are scared of what might happen between ourselves and our patients and not without reason. A high degree of integrity is required to work effectively in a way that truly combines the psyche with the soma.

The role of the remedy

I want to move on now to consider how the analytic concepts of projection and containment may be used to help articulate the role of the remedy in the evocation of certain placebo factors that are specific to homoeopathy.

I will be arguing:

- that the homoeopathic remedy is uniquely placed to contain projected impulses, experiences and feelings that otherwise might make their appearance as symptoms
- that the homoeopathic process of potentization is analogous to the therapist's detoxification of those impulses
- that the swallowing of the remedy is analogous to the patient's introjection of the therapist's capacity to contain previously toxic phenomena, and that this can contribute to symptom relief.

I will be looking for evidence from the case of Mrs A for the occurrence of these processes.

A dream

The night after first taking her Sepia, Mrs A reported waking from the following dream feeling nauseous with an aggravation of her backache.

My naughty 8-year-old son was in the car playing with the handbrake. I pulled him out of the car and thrashed him. Then I woke up.

There are a number of things that could be said about this short dream.

First, Levitan (1983) reports a series of dreams from people waking into asthma attacks. He found that such dreams tend to exhibit undisguised images of violence or sexual perversion. It is as if the dreamers have not quite succeeded in containing feelings or impulses sufficiently well to represent them symbolically in the dream in a disguised form. As a result they have woken up, and the uncontained conflict has precipitated symptoms. Perhaps Mrs A was on a similar threshold between symptom production and symbolic containment with this dream.

Secondly, like most dreams reported in the course of any treatment, this one is amenable to a transference/countertransference interpretation. It could be looked on as saying that if I were to get overexcited by Mrs A's flirtation with me, I could find myself in the position of the naughty son in the countertransference. His play with the phallic handbrake would then mirror my own, and the therapeutic relationship (car) would be in danger of crashing. On the other hand if I were to react too coldly to Mrs A's erotic play with me, she could find herself in the position of the child, with myself as the punitive mother. Morality would then be upheld, but only by leaving her with feelings of humiliation. This interpretation offers some confirmation of the existence of the erotic elements within the transference/countertransference postulated above.

The dream is amenable to another interpretation, however, if we regard her son as representing the needy dependent side of herself. It would then be bringing the way she attacks that part of herself to light. This interpretation is in line with my earlier speculation that Mrs A tended to cope with the stress of being unsupported in a strange country by violently suppressing her own needs. And her developing awareness of the cruelty with which she treated that part of herself may have helped diminish the severity of the attacks. This in turn could have contributed to the improvement in symptoms, such as the disturbance in appetite and digestive problems, which related to those attacks. The two interpretations above need not be mutually exclusive.

What consciously concerned Mrs A about her dream, though, were not these relatively deep unconscious processes, but the ferocity of her feelings towards her actual son. 'I did not realize how angry I was with him; my mother used to hit me, but I never hit my children' she said, in tears, in her next session. There was distress but also some relief at this recognition of feelings she had previously denied in herself. It would not be surprising if her experience of being hit by her mother had been so distressing that she had vowed never to inflict the same cruelty on her own children. And it may have been in order to achieve this goal that she had systematically 'misrecognized' her own feelings. At any rate, she was shocked to learn that the 'irritation' she thought she felt towards her son had turned out to be a towering rage.

This unrecognized rage could easily have contributed to most of her symptoms especially if we bear in mind that her son may have represented parts of herself as well as her actual son. The upper-backache that she had woken into could for instance have been brought on by rage locked into muscles as she tried to push it from consciousness (see Mr X). The nausea could have been an expression of her difficulty in digesting the fact that she had such violent gut feelings—a wish to vomit them out, and so on. Her recognition of these feelings seemed to help relieve these symptoms, and she reported a general improvement a few days after the dream that continued after the above session. The distress of her symptoms had in effect been replaced by the distress of consciously recognizing her conflicting feelings. This may not seem like much of a gain, but at least a dialogue had begun to open up between the different parts of herself where previously there had been a tyranny of the ego over the others.

This systematic misrecognition of feelings is something that has been commented on over the years by numerous analytic writers. It forms the basis of a famous paper on the 'mirror stage' by the French analyst Jacques Lacan (1949) for instance. It could even be said to underlie the very concept of the unconscious itself. It is safe to assume therefore that Mrs A is not alone in suffering symptoms as a result of denial of feelings. What is surprising though is that homoeopaths with their notion of disease coming from the 'inner person' have generally not made use of it. On the whole, Western medicine has been so successful at treating physical diseases that people who consult homoeopaths (and other complementary practitioners) tend to do so because they sense there is a significant psychological component to their suffering. Understanding the role of Mrs A's sepia in raising her conflicts from symptom to consciousness via the dream could therefore help to shed some more general light on the placebo effect within homoeopathy.

The remedy and dream formation

Such homoeopaths as Twentyman (1989) and Whitmont (1950) have written much on the origins of the remedy Sepia. It comes from cuttlefish ink, and this ink is released in a cloud when the animal is attacked. It seems to loom in the water acting as both a threat and a decoy to the predator while the vulnerable cuttlefish escapes. These writers have likened this inky cloud to the defensive eruption of the Sepia patient's anger, and these and other observations about Sepia are certainly pertinent to Mrs A.

According to homoeopathic theory, Sepia in its crude form should be capable of producing the symptoms from which Mrs A was suffering. This would include physical as well as emotional disturbances such as eruptions of anger with her nearest and dearest. The 'provings' from which the Sepia symptom picture was originally derived involved subjects knowingly taking material doses of Sepia and then reporting their subjective and objective observations (although the very first proving is said to have been an accidental one by an artist that Hahnemann the founder of homoeopathy was asked to treat). None of the early homoeopathic provings was double blind, though, so it is not clear which symptoms may have been produced by physical means and which by psychological means such as suggestion and association.

The Sepia that Mrs A took, like most homoeopathic remedies, had been 'potentized'. That is, it had been diluted and vigorously shaken to render it non-toxic while apparently retaining its medicinal power. It has been a long-standing mystery that the more dilute (potentized) the remedies the more powerfully they appear to act. Note, however, that the higher-potency medicines are given only when there is a precise fit between the remedy and the patient's symptom picture. Mrs A's symptom picture matched well with that of her remedy, and so a high-potency remedy was given.

If Mrs A knew much about the action of Sepia she would have consciously believed she was taking a detoxified version of a substance that could produce eruptions of anger. In this case it is easy to see how taking the remedy might then have the effect of helping her contain that anger. It would be a concrete equivalent of the internalization of the therapist's capacity to contain and detoxify dangerous elements within the transference/countertransference we saw earlier. Such an internalization might initiate a process of containment that allowed the unconscious rage to become conscious first in the dream, and then following a period of reflection, in the session. The rage had then come to express itself symbolically rather than symptomatically. She could now contain it.

There is little problem in understanding how the remedy might come to represent elements of experience detoxified within the therapeutic relationship such as Mrs A's sexual feelings. This could happen by simple association because taking the remedy reminded her of experiences in the session. And it is interesting to note in this connection that the sexual metaphors in her dream were more disguised than the violence—as if they had been more effectively worked through already.

How though could the remedy have helped her contain her largely unconscious violent rage if she didn't know the nature of Sepia? There could of course be a physical message carried in the remedy in some way at present unknown to science. But there is also a possible psychological explanation. The patient as we have seen comes to the homoeopath with a misrecognition of what she feels, and this produces symptoms. In Mrs A's case there is on the one hand a split between her ego and her rage. On the other hand she comes with the expectation or at least the hope of healing those symptoms. That is, she hopes to be made whole. She is unable to achieve this herself because the process would involve unbearable anxiety associated with shattering the image of who she wants to be. This in turn is associated in her case with feelings about being hit by her mother. The potential to heal is therefore projected on to the homoeopath, who is thus attributed with the power to perceive her rage despite her denial of it. She unconsciously believes his prescription must be of a substance that can produce rage in a crude dose. Every time she takes the remedy she is effectively taking in a detoxified version of that rage. This amounts to a message on a pill of milk sugar that says gently 'look, you're not like that, you're like this.' By the time she is able actually to dream of thrashing her son she has begun to accept that message consciously. As she continues to think about the dream and tell it to me, the process of symbolization and containment proceeds and symptom relief eventually follows. This explanation makes sense of my observation over the years, and confirmed by colleagues, that an effective homoeopathic remedy is often followed by an aggravation and a powerful but disturbing dream.

It also seems to make sense of the observation mentioned earlier that high-potency remedies appear to be the most effective. According to this view it is not so much the process of potentization that makes them effective. It is more the fact that the high potencies are prescribed when there is an especially good fit between the remedy and the patient's symptom picture. This 'good fit' is the equivalent of 'effective containment' for the patient's denied psychic contents, which are now projected into the remedy. All that needs to happen for this containment to occur is that patients accurately convey all their physical and emotional symptoms and also believe the homoeopath has found a remedy that effectively matches these. Their unconscious knowledge of the origin of their symptoms can then return to consciousness with the remedy in so far as they are ready and able to accept it. No doubt the homoeopath's confidence in his prescription conveys itself in such a case as well, reducing the patient's anxiety, and helping with the process.

CONCLUSION

In this chapter I have attempted to articulate some of the psychological factors that may contribute to the operation of the placebo effect in complementary medicine. In order to do this, I have applied some of the insights of psychoanalysis to the practice of acupuncture and homoeopathy. I have drawn in particular on two cases from my early work as a complementary practitioner. In both cases I hope to have shown how certain aspects of the transference and countertransference affected the outcome of treatment. These considerations, I would argue, have implications for understanding the operation of the placebo effect in most forms of medicine.

As well as these general considerations regarding transference and countertransference, I have attempted to use the language of psychoanalysis to help articulate some of the placebo factors that may be specific to homoeopathic medicine. In particular I have made use of the concepts of projection, containment and detoxification to explore how a homoeopathic remedy may help raise toxic-symptom-producing material into consciousness where it can eventually be more effectively contained. I have illustrated this paying particular attention to the function of dreaming in a particular case. But I hope the more general implications of that case will not be entirely lost to readers.

If this chapter has demonstrated that it can be fruitful to apply the tools of psychoanalysis to an exploration of the placebo effect, then it will have accomplished its task. I hope others will enjoy continuing that exploration.

REFERENCES

Alexander F 1950 Psychosomatic medicine. Norton, New York
Balint M 1957 The doctor the patient and his illness. Pitman Medical, London
Bateman A, Holmes J 1995 Introduction to psychoanalysis, contemporary theory and practice. Routledge, London
Bion W 1962 Learning from experience. Heinemann, Oxford
Eichenbaum, Orbach S 1985 Understanding women. Pelican, London
Foucault M 1970 The order of things. Random House, New York
Freud S 1893 Studies on hysteria, in the case of Anna Row. In: Collected works, standard edn, vol II. Hogarth, London, pp 21–48
Freud S 1914 Remembering repeating and working through. In: Collected works, standard edn, vol XII. Hogarth, London, p 151
Lacan J 1949 The mirror stage. In: Sheridan A (transl.) 1977 Ecrits a selection. Tavistock, London, pp 1–8
Levitan H L 1983 Dreams which precipitate asthma attacks. In: Krakowski A J, Kimble C P (eds) Psychosomatic medicine: theoretical, clinical and transcultural aspects. Plenum, New York, pp 79–87
Pietroni P 1989 Books reconsidered (the doctor his patient and the illness: Michael Balint). British Journal of Psychiatry 155:134–138
Samuels A 1993 The political psyche. Routledge, London
Twentyman R 1989 The science and art of healing. Floris, Edinburgh
Watkins A (ed) 1997 Mind–body medicine: a clinician's guide to psychoneuroimmunology. Churchill Livingstone, New York
Weiner H 1977 Psychobiology and human disease. Elsevier, New York
Whitmont E 1950 Sepia—analysis of dynamic totality. British Homoeopathic Journal XL (3):165
Wittgenstein L 1958 Philosophical investigations. Blackwell, Oxford

8

Intersubjectivity and the therapeutic relationship

Janet Richardson

Editor's note

Everyday clinical work leaves us in no doubt that practitioners who can create a therapeutic relationship add value to the therapeutic process. Nowhere is the contact between practitioner and patient more intense, prolonged and intimate than in nursing. We can understand then why so many writers in this field have thought about the therapeutic relationship. Nurses have also been at the forefront of a mainstream resurgence in touch-based therapies; many thousands of nurses in the UK have learned these approaches. Janet Richardson embodies all these concerns through her work in nursing development and teaching. At the time of writing she is also Chair of the Research Council for Complementary Medicine and recently based her doctoral thesis on an evaluation of the NHS Complementary Therapies Unit she helped set up for the Lewisham Hospital Trust in south-east London. Her chapter, exploring the overlap between nursing theory, touch, the therapeutic relationship and complementary therapies, indicates their common concern for a capacity to generate a 'shared space'. Practitioners from all fields will have their own experiences of shared consciousness and empathic moments; Janet's examples are from nursing and she sees them through the lens of nursing theory. Seeking to understand ways of optimizing what she calls 'the healing relationship', she highlights skilled use of narrative, empathy and openness. Janet sees them all as ways to create what she calls 'shared space' and she leaves open the question of whether this is just a metaphor for good communication or a state of being where the inner worlds of patient and practitioner actually interpenetrate.

It is my intention in this chapter to explore the idea that the effect commonly referred to as the 'placebo effect' could be, in part, a therapeutic process arising from an experience that is essentially intersubjective. In order to do this I will explore theoretical perspectives of intersubjectivity that are grounded in psychology and nursing. Where possible, the theoretical approaches will be supported by research evidence. More importantly, however, I will include examples from clinical practice that illustrate this view of 'shared consciousness' or intersubjective experience. The ideas in this chapter have developed from my own background and understanding of psychology, and my experience of nursing theories and clinical practice.

THEORETICAL APPROACHES THAT SUPPORT AN INTERSUBJECTIVE SCIENCE

Much of 'medical' care is aimed at the exploration of physical/biological processes in order to understand and treat diseased bodies (and to some extent diseased minds). We examine 'objective' measures of disease and seek 'objective' outcome measures in order to monitor our treatment successes. This objectivist paradigm currently dominates Western medicine and science. For example it is a commonly held view in psychology that perceptions are private and 'subjective' and that physical objects are public and 'objective' (Velmans 2000a). This view colours the way we think of and interpret private experiences and physical objects. We assign greater importance to physical events as they can be observed 'objectively'; feelings and experiences can (only) be reported by the experiencer. Consider, however, the importance given to research into pain (a subjective experience) and its management, with over 148 000 publications listed on the Medline database (Velmans 2000a). Velmans presents a persuasive reanalysis of private versus public phenomena:

Each (private) observation or experience is necessarily *subjective*, in that it is always the observation or experience of a *given* observer, viewed and described from his or her individual perspective. However, once that experience is shared with another observer it can become *intersubjective* ... To the extent that an experience or observation can be *generally* shared (by a community of observers), it can form part of the data-base of a communal science.

This approach suggests the possibility of an intersubjective science in which our phenomenal worlds can be rigorously explored and interpreted.

The potential application of an intersubjective science to a clinical setting is interesting. Indeed there is a strong tradition within nursing of studying the 'lived experience' of illness through the methodology of interpretive phenomenology (Benner 1994a). In this method 'the interpretive researcher creates a dialogue between practical concerns and lived experience through engaged reasoning and imaginative dwelling in the immediacy of the participants' worlds' (Benner 1994b). Benner (1994b) suggests that nurses are well suited to phenomenology as they are accustomed to 'getting the person's story'. Interpretive phenomenologists apply a range of skills to their research that are completely conducive to a therapeutic encounter: open listening, active listening and allowing the interviewee to shape the telling of the story. In order to interpret the data the researcher is required to move into the phenomenal world of the participant.

It is possible to see how this approach can be used to understand and interpret the experience of illness through subjective reports that contribute to intersubjective data. For example we might be able to report the 'objective' blood gases of patients who have chronic obstructive airways disease, but we could also report that patients who have this condition make sense of it in terms of fighting a battle and 'going to war' (O'Callaghan, unpublished work, 1998).

THE PATIENT ASSESSMENT: PROCESS, RESEARCH AND CLINICAL PRACTICE

History taking

For a practitioner, the first point of contact with a patient involves taking a history. Though essentially a fact-finding enterprise, the history taking is (potentially) the beginning of the therapeutic relationship. During this initial period of questioning, practitioners' response (or lack of response) to patients' answers and subtle cues, such as facial expression and body language, will demonstrate their skills in 'active listening'. When patients consciously (or unconsciously) process the practitioners' responses, they will adjust their participation in this process, appropriately elaborating or restricting their answers to the questions. Taking a history is rather like encouraging people to tell a story, their personal story. However, in health-care we often expect patients to tell their story in a way that is tightly ordered and structured so that we can make sure that we have not missed something important, such as a family history of high blood pressure.

We expect the patient's story to be told in a language that is familiar to us, in 'clinical language', so that we can order all the facts, recognize a pattern and prescribe appropriate treatment. This process is particularly important for junior and inexperienced staff who have not fully assimilated all the relevant questions into their natural repertoire. However, this approach to taking a patient's history can easily interrupt the flow of the narrative; for example Beckman & Frankel (1984) found that patients were interrupted by their doctors approximately 18 seconds after they began to speak. In contrast, excellent physicians 'are those who spend time with the patient and thereby gain an understanding of both the clinical problem and the patient's life situation' (Landau 1993). The form of questioning used in taking a 'medical history' attempts to identify symptom patterns in order to detect the presence or absence of 'disease'. In contrast 'illness' refers to how sick people and their wider social network respond to symptoms and disability. This latter approach could be described as the 'lived experience' of bodily processes (symptoms) such as respiratory wheezes and painful joints (Kleinman 1988).

The illness experience and its meaning

It is the *illness experience* that may be overlooked in our attempts to record and categorize symptoms. Experience of illness includes an explanation of that experience in common-sense ways that are accessible to lay persons within the patient's social group and culture, and the extent to which the problems and distress impact on their everyday lives. *Disease* is what practitioners are trained to see, so they reconfigure the patient's problems as narrow, technical problems, and are unconcerned with patients' narratives and causal beliefs (Kleinman 1988). For the patient illness also has *meaning*; yet (biomedical) healthcare is organized in order to pursue the biological mechanisms of disease, and to avoid the exploration of the illness experience and its meaning.

The meaning associated with an illness will depend on social and cultural factors, but also the limitations and trajectory of the illness. So for example elderly patients experiencing postoperative pain following a total hip replacement might interpret the pain as necessary for healing. They might expect that it will be of short duration, followed by increased mobility and the absence of the chronic pain they have suffered for the past 2 years or more. In contrast, patients experiencing pain following a mastectomy for the removal of a malignant tumour might wonder if this is the kind of pain they can expect to experience for the rest of their life. They will be concerned about the results of the histology, that the cancer may have spread more widely than was originally thought, that it might recur, and how they will cope with their family and young children? The pain takes on a sinister meaning associated with uncertainty, possible future suffering and, ultimately, possible death from the cancer.

Through detailed inquiry and active listening the practitioner can enter the patient's phenomenal world of illness. Kleinman (1988) proposes a clinical method for the care of the chronically sick. This involves the 'empathic witnessing' of the experience of suffering through sensitively facilitating patients to tell their story of the illness.

Consider the case study in Box 9.1, which is an example taken from clinical practice.

Box 9.1   Case study 1

A woman presents to an NHS complementary therapy clinic for acupuncture treatment. She has been referred by her general practitioner with a clinical problem of 'chronic low-back pain'. She is 54 years of age, she has had her back problem for 8 years and has been treated with a variety of methods: bed rest, traction, physiotherapy, and non-steroidal anti-inflammatory drugs. She is also under the care of the orthopaedic team. The patient has no experience of acupuncture and is somewhat nervous and apprehensive about the consultation.

The acupuncturist begins to take a detailed history asking questions that are unfamiliar to the patient. It becomes apparent during the history taking that the patient is also suffering from a frozen shoulder. The patient noticeably begins to relax; this is clearly a consultation where she is being taken seriously and the acupuncturist is taking time in listening to her history. The acupuncturist then asks a further question: 'How did you come to have this pain?' The patient draws a deep breath and says 'you are the first person to ask me that'; she then begins to weep. This is clearly an important moment in the consultation and the acupuncturist holds that moment and gently begins to explore it with the patient: 'Perhaps you would like to tell me about it?' At this point the patient reveals her own story. When her son was 7 years old he started to have fits. The GP suggested that these were not serious and that the boy would grow out of them. But the fits got worse, and no investigations were performed until he suffered some limb paralysis at the age of 19. Finally a brain scan revealed an inoperable tumour. Distraught and angry, our patient decided to care for her son at home. This she did until he died. However, she was unaware of the range of possible services that could have supported her in this home care, and they were never offered. Consequently she struggled with the physical care, which involved lifting and moving her son who was by then aged 21. This, so she believes, resulted in physical damage to her back. The emotional care, the love and concern for her son, and her own distress, were intertwined with her anger towards medical staff. Her physical and emotional state were still unresolved after 8 years of 'treatment'*.

The outcome for this patient was positive. She was treated with a course of acupuncture, but only after she had been given the time and space during which she could tell her story to someone completely present for her. After three treatments her frozen shoulder greatly improved and by the time she was discharged following her sixth treatment her physical problems were much improved. But in addition she had moved on emotionally to a place from which she could begin the lengthy process of healing.

* This case (history) is presented to the reader as it was presented to the practitioner by the patient. It is not my intention to draw any conclusions or make any judgements about the professional management of the patient's son.

A discussion with the practitioner following that first consultation revealed an interesting phenomena. The practitioner reported how she experienced the emotional distress and anger experienced by the patient, and felt the physical tension of the patient's back problem in her own back. The practitioner was also consciously aware that in allowing the patient to tell her story and share her distress, and in honouring the story, the 'healing space' the patient had been denied in previous treatments could be created. It was the practitioner's opinion that if the patient had not been able to unpack her story in that first consultation she would still have a chronic back problem.

King (1990) provides an operational definition of 'space' as follows. Space exists in all directions, is the same everywhere, and is defined by the physical area known as 'territory' and by the behaviours of those who occupy it. Space is characterized as universal, but may be personal, subjective, situational or dependent on relationships in the situation, or based on the individual's perception of the situation (George 1995a).

In Newman's theory, 'space' is discussed in conjunction with time and movement on the basis of the following relationships (see George 1995b):

- time and space have a complementary relationship
- movement is a means by which space and time become reality
- movement is a reflection of consciousness
- time is a function of movement
- time is a measurement of consciousness.

The notion of 'space' in the context of an intersubjective science is explored more fully in Richardson (2000).

EMPATHY AND INTERSUBJECTIVITY IN CLINICAL PRACTICE

Empathy

The process described above might be interpreted as a form of empathy. The concept of empathy is fundamental to the healing relationship and could be defined as 'respect for and openness to the concerns of the patient and her family' (Levasseur & Vance 1993). Though empathy can clearly be used as a specific and conscious intervention, it is also possible that some of the positive outcomes of therapeutic interventions that are due to so called non-specific (placebo) effects may be due to the practitioner's mobilization of empathy, on either a conscious or unconscious level. Empathy is a fundamental underpinning of the therapeutic relationship in counselling and psychotherapy. It involves 'entering the private perceptual world of the other and becoming thoroughly at home in it' (Rogers 1975).

Halpern (1993) refers to clinical empathy as an emotional resonance where the goal is to understand in a detailed and experiential way what the patient is feeling, and suggests that this requires emotional engagement. The ability of a therapist to empathize and 'be with' a patient may, however, be constrained by that therapist's own fears and anxieties. For example Jacobs (1989) reports:

I may not like what a patient is doing. I may be angry. But I try to keep these feelings against a background of the overall dialogic attitude that I am maintaining. This dialogic attitude is often not communicated in words, really; it develops over time, and is more often sustained by non-verbal behaviour or by tone of voice than by any words spoken. In a few instances recently, when I confronted patients in my anger, I could really feel my ability to be with the patients in my anger and still be open and receptive to them. The vibrancy of the meetings was remarkable. This was very different from times when I have set limits out of my own frustration, been psychologically cut off from the patient's experiences, and wanted them to do something to make me feel better.

Storytelling

It is possible to develop empathy through the exploration of the patient's narrative. Through narrative knowledge 'humans come to recognize themselves and each other, telling stories in order to know who they are' (Charon 1993). Much of the work of the clinician involves listening to patients' stories and making sense of their accounts of illness and how individual and family lives are affected. Charon suggests that it is only with narrative competence that a clinician can deliver empathic care. (Also see Ch. 8.)

Stories play a major part in our lives as human beings, and we need to be able to tell them (Gersie 1997). In predominantly oral traditions they are the main mode of transmission for important information such as traditional practices, rituals, the use of medicinal substances and cultural history. We construct our world and who we are through stories, stories about childhood, what we did on holiday, how we came to be in the job we are in, how we met our partner and fell in love. All our stories are expressions of ourselves and are necessary to 'weave a web of meaning within which we can live'. They provide the context of normality within which we live our lives (Mair 1989). Storytelling is a way of placing life changes and rites of passage in a mythical and wider cultural context.

Stories not only provide context and meaning to our lives, they can be a tangible way of sharing thoughts and feelings that, in 'normal' conversation, we feel unable to express. By placing our experiences in a mythical and imaginative context, particularly in times of pain and distress, it is possible to express and explore that distress in a profound and deeply meaningful way (see for example Mellon 1992). Storymaking can be an important therapeutic activity for example in dealing with life changes, loss and bereavement (Gersie 1991, 1997, Gersie & King 1990).

Storytelling also serves the healing professions very well. We write case studies for professional journals in order to communicate new findings in treatments and healthcare practices, we present 'cases' to colleagues that tell a story about a normal or unusual 'picture' of a 'disease'. But we also tell stories about 'patients', communicating their courage and understanding in the context of their illness (see for example Lynn 1993, Remen 1996). Such stories, communicated beautifully and with profound respect, capture the qualities and depths of the human condition, which during the course of our lives we inevitably encounter.

Studies of different psychotherapeutic models suggest that there is little difference in outcome between contrasting therapeutic orientations (Barkham 1992). However, therapist variables appear to exert a strong influence on therapeutic outcome irrespective of theoretical orientation

(Barkham 1992, Norcross & Arkowitz 1992). The quality of the therapeutic relationship can provide a space in which patients are able to tell their story, and foster the feeling that their story matters (Schreiber 1996). This storytelling and listening process enables an exploration of meaning, or the redefining of meaning, and this in itself may provide a therapeutic outcome (Charlton 1991, Mair 1997).

Through the process of listening to and telling stories it is possible for individuals to move into a shared space, where time seems to stand still and the boundaries between self and other appear to merge. (For example in my training in transpersonal counselling skills this 'space' was described as: the moment when the dialogue between counsellor and client becomes a dance, and the room seems to disappear. See also Ch. 7.) Where the distinctions between the storyteller and the listener dissolve, there is only the presence of the story.

Engagement in therapeutic relationships

Consider Figure 9.1. This diagram is reproduced from a chapter by Velmans (1998) in a book on virtual realities. It is pictorial representation of a dream (mine), in which people are enclosed in bubbles that are virtual

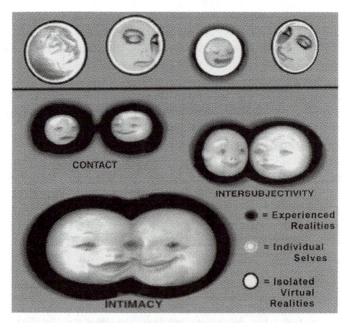

Figure 9.1   Experienced realities: intersubjectivity in relationships. (Drawn by John Wood. From Velmans M 1998 Psychological, physical, and virtual realities. In: Wood J The virtual embodied. Routledge, London. Reproduced with permission.)

worlds. Whilst people are enclosed in their virtual worlds they may engage in relationship but there is no genuine contact between them. In intersubjectivity, however, the boundaries of the bubbles become semipermeable, there is genuine engagement and openness to each other, and this is the space in which empathy can exist.

Perhaps you have observed consultations where the patient and practitioner appear to be communicating, but no real engagement is taking place? Such practitioners are 'in their head', taking in facts, working through patterns (under time pressure), and making notes, but are not really engaged in the process. Consequently in their lack of engagement they miss vital cues that are not followed through. They also communicate to the patient that they are only seeking answers to their questions and do not require full elaboration (the patient's story). You will also no doubt remember consultations you have witnessed that look something very like the intersubjectivity picture—where both patient and practitioner are fully present in the consultation, sharing the experience from their relative perspectives.

The themes of 'openness' and 'engagement' are explored in detail in a number of nursing theories (Newman 1994, Rogers 1992). In these theories human beings are described as 'unitary' beings who are 'open' in their interaction with their environment; there are no real boundaries between individual and environment (George 1995a).

In developing her theory, Newman drew on physicist David Bohm's discussion on implicate and explicate order and Moss's presentation of love as the highest level of consciousness (George 1995b). For Newman, disease is a meaningful reflection of the whole and health is 'expanding consciousness'. Newman sees health as a 'pattern of the whole within a normal progression toward higher levels of organisation'. These 'open energy systems' described by Newman appear to be similar to the picture representing intersubjectivity in Figure 9.1. Newman suggests that the open energy systems are in constant interaction, influencing one another's patterns as they evolve together. Thus an individual's dis-ease relates to and affects the patterns of others (George 1995b). This particular approach suggests that the separation of *self* and *other* is not as clearly defined as we might imagine (or hope!), and that the manifestation of 'openness' and 'engagement' may be a product of how aware we are of *self*, and the relationship of *self* to *other*.

BEING PRESENT AND THE HEALING EFFECT

If we follow through Newman's theory of interacting open energy systems and 'patterns' of expanding consciousness, it is possible to see similarities between her theory and the role of empathy and 'presence' in the therapeutic relationship. Indeed Newman (1994) states that the intention of

---

Box 9.2 Case study 2

A clinical nurse specialist in acute pain is called to assess a patient. The patient is recovering from major surgery she had 2 days earlier. She also has an unrelated chronic pain problem that had not been fully assessed or treated prior to surgery. The nurse assesses the patient who is clearly in severe pain even at rest. A further pain-killing drug exhausts what is available on the drug chart and the anaesthetist is called to revise the medication. While awaiting the anaesthetist the nurse realizes that she shares the patient's feelings of helplessness. Remembering what little she knows about Therapeutic Touch she suggests to the patient that providing gentle support for her head might be useful. Then removing the back of the bed and the pillows, the nurse gently cradles the patient's head, focusing her intention on supporting and being with the patient. When asked why she did this she later reported 'I felt as if I was experiencing the patient's pain and distress and there was nothing I could do but be there'. She explained that she recalled that Therapeutic Touch could be used as a way of communicating with patients, particularly when 'there was nothing I could *say* that would help'.

---

nursing is to: 'enter into the process with the client to be present with it and live it, even if it appears in the form of disharmony, catastrophe, or disease'.

Rowan (1998) suggests a therapeutic relationship that 'goes beyond empathy' and is similar to that described by Newman. He calls this 'linking' and describes a process by which another person's world overlaps with our own world, whereby practitioners can be with patients from the inside and share their subjective experience. Robbins (1998) also describes a process that he suggests is a form of 'therapeutic presence', which requires openness and awareness of the intersubjective space between therapist and patient: 'In order to understand an experience, I must first feel its contours, touch the very texture of its existence, and take the substance of the interaction into my body'.

It is interesting to note that over 30 years ago nurses were advised to 'get inside the skin' of their patients in order to know what they need (Henderson 1960). The case study in Box 9.2 is a lovely example of a brief moment of this demonstrated in clinical practice.

Touch

Nurses frequently use touch as a means of communication and to provide comfort to patients who are in pain or distressed (Sayer-Adams & Wright 1995). Physical contact between nurse and patient may take place in different contexts and for different reasons. The physical contact may contribute to a therapeutic outcome, though this is likely to be determined by the nature and purpose of the contact, and the intent of the nurse. For example 'instrumental touch' is the deliberate physical contact made as part of a procedure, such as the dressing of a wound, whereas 'expressive touch', such as a hug to comfort a patient or relative, is a demonstration of concern and support. In contrast, 'Therapeutic Touch' (see Ch. 11) involves mobilizing the *intent* of the nurse and the transferring of 'energy' in order to produce a positive therapeutic effect (Tutton 1991). Our awareness of *self* and our own personal stories will no doubt influence and empower our intent—that is, our ability to utilize *intention* therapeutically in the context of a healthcare relationship. Whether one is consciously using touch as a therapeutic intervention or providing some form of psychotherapeutic action in the context of nursing, it appears that there is something about the quality of the relationship and the quality of 'presence' that is important in the therapeutic interaction (Ersser 1991). (The role of intention in Therapeutic Touch is discussed in further detail by Wright & Sayre-Adams in Ch. 11.)

The healing relationship

Benner (1984) demonstrates through phenomenological research how a healing relationship between a patient and a nurse can positively affect the therapeutic outcome or the ability of the patient to deal with life-threatening illness. Benner provides examples of how a healing relationship, using therapeutic goals and intentions, can help patients to change their behaviour, 'helping them to become more social and cultural beings who can interact more satisfyingly with other people'. In contrast to the dominance of cure in medicine, Benner's work emphasizes the caring and empowering work of nursing and shows how this can have profound effects on patients' physical, social and emotional well-being.

Benner's research of 'novice' and 'expert' nurses shows that several steps occur in the development of the healing relationship. The first, mobilizing hope for the nurse and the patient, requires the nurse to recognize that the patient has the capacity of making positive life changes and then to make a conscious decision to help this; thus the patient's sense of hope is mobilized. The second step is where the nurse helps the patient to find an acceptable interpretation or understanding of the illness, pain, fear, anxiety or other stressful emotion. In the third step the nurse assists the patient to use appropriate social, emotional or spiritual support.

Once the healing relationship is established, subtle interventions and ways of 'being with' a patient appear to make a positive difference in recovery—for example the provision of comfort measures and 'preserving personhood' in the face of pain and extreme breakdown. Such skills are predominantly found in expert rather than novice nurses (Benner 1984). This expert behaviour emerges out of a (personal) way of being, and of being in relation to others. The concept of *doing to* a patient is prevalent in Western medicine, whereas the notion of *being with* is little practised let alone understood. What Benner describes as 'presencing', is, on the surface, simply staying with the patient during a time of pain, discomfort or loss. It is, however, a form of communication that requires little verbal activity and is, to a large extent, dependent on nurses' own emotional/spiritual development and their sense of humanness.

This healing and caring approach taken by nurses could be defined as empathy, presencing or intersubjectivity. It has been eloquently described by Henderson (1960) as follows: 'The nurse is temporarily the consciousness of the unconscious, the love of the life of the suicidal, the legs of the amputee, the eyes of the newly blind, the means of locomotion for the infant, knowledge and confidence for the young mother, the voice for those too weak or withdrawn to speak'.

SYNTHESIS: THE RELATIONSHIP OF RESEARCH AND THEORY TO CLINICAL PRACTICE

Healing models

There is little doubt that the ability of the practitioner to create a 'healing space' and therapeutic relationship with a patient can influence the therapeutic process. Hodges & Scofield (1995) propose a 'healing model' as a primary mechanism underlying much of conventional and complementary medicine. This model incorporates many of the factors thought to bring about a placebo response, in particular the role of the therapeutic relationship. It is then possible to conceptualize a 'healing effect' potentially underlying and contributing to *all* forms of therapeutic intervention. Given the power of this effect, it might be more useful to view it positively rather than be dismissive: to attempt to mobilize it for the benefit of the patient.

Frank (1984) examined similarities between psychotherapy and placebo effects in medicine and suggested that some of the basic ingredients in all therapies include: arousing hope, emotional arousal, encouraging changed activity and encouraging new ways of understanding oneself and one's problems. Benner (1984) found that arousing hope was the first step in the development of the healing relationship in nursing. Frank (1984) suggested that the following therapeutic components were shared by different psychotherapeutic models: a confiding relationship with a helping person, a healing setting, a conceptual scheme or myth to explain symptoms, and a ritual to help resolve symptoms. These therapeutic components are clearly common to all therapeutic relationships from Western medical interventions to shamanic interventions (Helman 1990, Kakar 1982).

Use of narrative

It may be possible to mobilize 'healing' factors by attending to patient expectations, the provision of good quality information, the use of deep relaxation (or hypnosis) and of distraction techniques. Perhaps fundamental to all these activities is the power of the relationship between patient and practitioner. Our ability as practitioners to work with narrative, to hear the story and be open to the suffering is a good place to start. The healing process may begin in that point of focus and shared consciousness (or intersubjectivity) where patients feel that their experience is deeply understood, and therefore their personhood is valued.

Charon (1993) suggests several ways in which practitioners can be taught to improve their narrative competence.

- Writing from the patient's point of view, in particular when patient consultation has resulted in the practitioner feeling angry or frustrated, can be useful to think one's way into the patient's circumstances and feelings that may have contributed to the behaviour resulting in the practitioner's own frustration.
- Reading serious fiction can exercise narrative skills and expose the practitioner to other lives and realities. Charon also suggests reading some of the traditional stories, fairy tales and myths, as they often parallel our own lives and can help us to find meaning in difficult and distressing circumstances.
- Practitioners should recognize the way in which medicine strikes home—that 'clinical' judgements may be influenced by one's own experiences (e.g. practitioners' own unheard stories and unfinished business).

Narratives in research can reveal practices and concerns that are embedded in the social and moral culture of healthcare (Wros 1994). We can begin to understand 'what it is like' for our patients through the development of an 'intersubjective science': 'That is, through the sharing of a similar experience, subjective views and descriptions of that experience potentially converge, enabling intersubjective agreement about what has been experienced' (Velmans 1999).

For example an intersubjective science could focus research on illness rather than disease, such as attempting to understand what it is like to live with chronic illness (Benner et al 1994). This research approach, conducted within a rigorous methodological framework (see for example Benner 1994a, Velmans 2000b), is not simply about developing an interesting form of inquiry. It could facilitate the healing professions in understanding the patients' experience, so that they are able to help patients to live with their illness, find meaning and so on.

Healers' personal qualities

Perhaps our development as practitioners includes the process of empathy, the ability to 'be with' our patients, providing the 'presencing' that Benner (1984) refers to. If this quality of relationship can make important differences to therapeutic outcomes, these skills might need a more prominent place in the education of healthcare professionals. Katz (1963) suggests that, with discipline, empathy or 'empathic understanding' becomes a fully reputable scientific technique, and that when empathy is used in a professional way it becomes more consistently effective. Empathy requires openness. 'Caring requires that we be open', but it is also important to acknowledge that being open also requires us to be vulnerable (George 1995a). By focusing on our own openness (in the context of our relationships with patients), and being aware of our personal stress and limitations, we might be more able to affect a therapeutic process. This way of 'being with' and working with patients requires us to consider how we might retain appropriate vulnerability, whilst ensuring that our own personhood remains intact. One mechanism through which this vulnerability and openness can be contained is in relationship with another professional who acts as 'supervisor'. This is common practice for psychotherapists and counsellors, and is now a basic requirement in clinical nursing (clinical supervision).

Although it is possible, through research, to tease out some of the variables that contribute to a therapeutic outcome (over and above the 'active' intervention), the interaction of social, cultural and personal factors remain complex. It may, however, be possible that some practitioners are simply more 'therapeutic' than others. Needleman (1985) talks of the indefinable, yet instantly recognizable qualities that manifest when a practitioner is also a 'healer'. These 'indefinable' qualities may be grounded in an intersubjective process—that is, an ability to move, through the use of narrative, empathy and openness, into a shared (healing) space with the patient. This is a space in which the world of the patient overlaps with the world of the practitioner, a space in which the 'doing' is less important than the 'being'.

ACKNOWLEDGEMENTS

I would like to thank Jessica Darling (acupuncturist) and Karen Gardiner (clinical nurse specialist in acute pain) for sharing their cases studies with me, also Julie O'Callaghan for sharing her research.

REFERENCES

Barkham M 1992 Research on integrative and eclectic therapy. In: Dryden W (ed) Integrative and eclectic therapy: a handbook. Open University Press, Buckingham, UK
Beckman H, Frankel R 1984 Evaluation of humanistic qualities in the internist. Annals of Internal Medicine 99:720–724
Benner P 1984 From novice to expert: excellence and power in clinical nursing practice. Addison-Wesley, California
Benner P (ed) 1994a Interpretive phenomenology. Embodiment, caring and ethics in health and illness. Sage, Thousand Oaks ,CA

Benner P 1994b The tradition and skill of interpretive phenomenology in studying health, illness and caring. In: Benner P (ed) Interpretive phenomenology. Embodiment, caring and ethics in health and illness. Sage, Thousand Oaks, CA

Benner P, Janson-Bjerklie S, Ferketich S, Becker G 1994 Moral dimensions of living with a chronic illness. In: Benner P (ed) Interpretive phenomenology. Embodiment, caring and ethics in health and illness. Sage, Thousand Oaks, CA

Charlton B G 1991 Stories of sickness. British Journal of General Practice June: 222–223

Charon R 1993 The narrative road to empathy. In: Spiro H, Curnen M G, Peschel E, St James D (eds) Empathy and the practice of medicine. Yale University Press, New Haven, CT, pp 151-158

Ersser S 1991 A search for the therapeutic dimensions of nurse–patient interaction. In: McMahon R, Pearson A (eds) Nursing as therapy. Chapman & Hall, London, p 56

Frank J D 1984 Persuasion and healing: a comparative study of psychotherapy, 2nd edn. John Hopkins University Press, Baltimore, MD

George J B 1995a Imogene M King. In: George J B (ed) Nursing theories: the base for professional nursing practice, 4th edn. Prentice Hall, Englewood Cliffs, NJ, p 215

George J B 1995b Margaret Newman. In: George J B (ed) Nursing theories: the base for professional nursing practice, 4th edn. Prentice Hall, Englewood Cliffs, NJ, p 392

Gersie A 1991 Storymaking in bereavement: dragons flight in the meadow. Jessica Kingsley, London

Gersie A 1997 Reflections on therapeutic storymaking: the use of stories in groups. Jessica Kingsley, London

Gersie A, King N 1990 Storymaking in education and therapy. Jessica Kingsley, London

Halpern J 1993 Empathy: using resonance emotions in the service of curiosity. In: Spiro H, Curnen M G, Peschel E, St James D (eds) Empathy and the practice of medicine. Yale University Press, New Haven, CT, p 161

Helman C G 1990 Culture, health and illness, 2nd edn. Butterworth Heinemann, Oxford

Henderson V 1960 The basic principles of nursing care. International Council for Nurses, London

Hodges D, Scofield T 1995 The healing effect—complementary medicine's unifying principle? Network 58:3–8

Jacobs 1989 Dialogue in gestalt theory and therapy. Gestalt Journal 8(1):25–37

Kakar S 1982 Shamans, mystics and doctors. Mandala, London

Katz R L 1963 Empathy: its nature and uses. Free Press, New York

King I 1990 A theory for nursing: systems, concepts, process. Delmar, Albany, NY

Kleinman A 1988 The illness narratives: suffering, healing and the human condition. Basic Books, New York

Landau R L 1993 … And the least of these is empathy. In: Spiro H, Curnen M G, Peschel E, St James D (eds) Empathy and the practice of medicine. Yale University Press, New Haven, CT, p 108

Levasseur J, Vance D R 1993 Doctors, nurses and empathy. In: Spiro H, Curnen M G, Peschel E, St James D (eds) Empathy and the practice of medicine. Yale University Press, New Haven, CT, p 81

Lynn J 1993 Travels in the valley of the shadow. In: Spiro H, Curnen M G, Peschel E, St James D (eds) Empathy and the practice of medicine. Yale University Press, New Haven, CT, pp 41–47

Mair M 1989 Between psychology and psychotherapy: a poetics of experience. Routledge, London

Mair M 1997 Conversational inquiry: questioning our understanding. In: Richardson J, Velmans M (eds) Methodologies for the study of consciousness: a new synthesis. Proceedings of An International Symposium

Mellon N 1992 Storytelling and the art of imagination. Element, Shaftesbury, Dorset

Needleman J 1985 The way of the physician. Arkana, London

Newman M A 1994 Health as expanding consciousness, 2nd edn. National League for Nursing, NY

Norcross J C, Arkowitz H 1992 The evolution and current status of psychotherapy integration. In: Dryden W (ed) Integrative and eclectic therapy: a handbook. Open University Press, Buckingham, UK, pp 10–11

Remen R N 1996 Kitchen table wisdom. Pan, London

Richardson J 2000 Clinical implications of an intersubjective science. In: Velmans M (ed) Investigating consciousness: new methodologies and maps. John Benjamins, Amsterdam

Robbins A (ed) 1998 Therapeutic presence. Jessica Kingsley, London

Rogers C 1975 Empathic: an unappreciated way of being. Counselling Psychologist 5(2):2–10

Rogers M E 1992 Nursing science and the space age. Nursing Science Quarterly (5):27–34

Rowan J 1998 Linking: its place in therapy. International Journal of Psychotherapy 3(3):245–354

Sayer-Adams J, Wright S 1995 The theory and practice of therapeutic touch. Churchill Livingstone, New York

Schreiber R 1996 (Re)defining my self: women's process of recovery from depression. Qualitative Health Research 6:469–491

Tutton E 1991 An exploration of touch and its use in nursing. In: McMahon R, Pearson A (eds) Nursing as therapy. Chapman & Hall, New York, pp 144–147

Velmans M 1998 Physical, psychological and virtual realities. In: Wood J (ed) The virtual embodied: presence, practice, technology. Routledge, London

Velmans M 1999 Intersubjective science. Journal of Consciousness Studies 6 (2/3):299–306

Velmans M (2000a) Understanding consciousness. Routledge, London

Velmans M (ed) (2000b) Investigating consciousness: new methodologies and maps. John Benjamins, Amsterdam

Wros P L 1994 The ethical context of nursing care of dying patients in critical care. In: Benner P (ed) Interpretive phenomenology. Embodiment caring and ethics in health and illness. Sage, Thousand Oaks, CA, pp 266–272

Placebo responses in bodywork*

Phil Latey

Editor's note

For many years I have admired Phil's ability to think about osteopathic body work. He has an extraordinary ability to notice aspects of the consultation that most of us miss; and also a way of confronting his fellow practitioners with their own unexamined beliefs and assumptions. Phil brings a psychotherapist's sensitivities to the bodywork session, where he sees two embodied minds at work, each one entwined with its individual family and cultural history. His chapter explores the non-specific effects involved in manual therapies with their positive and negative potential. Phil raises two particularly fascinating possibilities, concerning undeniably non-specific elements in the consultation that are also substantial and literally tangible: in fact both can only be known through touch. One is the ability of the skilled psychologically aware bodyworker to help people re-embody themselves. The other is the extraordinary notion that subtle but powerful therapeutic effects may involve a kind of body-to-body entrainment. This is an experience many bodyworkers as well as psychotherapists would attest to; a more concrete version of Bob Wither's ideas that containment can be enacted through the ceremonial of complementary therapy and that they can trigger healing responses. In this chapter Lately takes us to the mysterious leading edge of conscious bodywork.

*This chapter is based on an article that first appeared in the *Journal of Bodywork and Movement Therapies* (Latey P 2000 Placebo: a study of persuasion and rapport. Journal of Bodywork and Movement Therapies 4(2): 123–136).

The reflections in this chapter come from 27 years of clinical experience in osteopathic private practice. For the most part my patients have been fee paying, and were referred by 'word of mouth' reputation. Some of that reputation has been gained through rapid and impressive successes; some has come through very long-term work with severe and intractable problems.

During my years of training at the British School of Osteopathy in London (BSO) between 1969 and 1972 I was convinced that many of the senior lecturers were without doubt extremely capable human 'horse whisperers'. They were reluctant to acknowledge how much this quality of persuasiveness contributed to their treatment. But I felt they nevertheless revealed that they were well aware that couchside manner was central to their success.

For us who work on our patients' bodies as osteopaths, the really hard question then as now is to decide how much of our real (or apparent) clinical effect is due to *placebo-like responses* and *persuasion*, how much to bodily changes directly attributable to *specific biomechanical elements* of the manual therapy, and how much might be due to other factors?

THE PLACEBO RESPONSE IN BODYWORK

In order to begin making clinical sense of this we need to make two useful basic distinctions:

- *placebo responsiveness*, which can be defined as attributable solely to the patient
- *persuasiveness*, which I would define as the combined effect of conscious and/or unconscious elements in the practitioner's clinical repertoire.

The thoughtful reader might argue—since touch and movement are more or less unconsciously meaningful—that many tactile and structural techniques could fall into this category. I would agree and therefore the differences between suggestion and clinical rapport *including its physicality* will be discussed later in the chapter.

It is not easy to study these qualities, and clearly they are precisely the sort of individual differences that the randomized clinical trial (RCT) is designed to exclude. Nor could such an experimental approach be either ethical (for how can the bodywork practitioner give 'dummy' treatments?) or practical (as though the practitioner could be wholly impersonal in his approach). And, since in reality our practices rely on patients being so strongly self-selecting (and therefore far from a random sample), the whole notion of using an RCT study falls apart even for the purpose of comparing groups of patients 'randomized' amongst various practitioners or therapies (see Ch. 12). Therefore, in attempting to study the non-specific elements at work in osteopathy, I am relying on my years of observation to make some predictions about the importance of certain factors.

Placebo responsiveness: patient factors

To me it seems that a great deal of placebo responsiveness can be predicted from the way patients come to their initial consultation. In the very short term these clues become strong predictors of our success rates with uncomplicated problems.

Favourable factors

Personal reputation contributes a lot to the favourable preconditions (Box 10.1). If patients have actually heard of our success and skills from two or more people, or even a whole social group who we have been looking after, this is strongly favourable. Also helpful are a set of expectations that fit with our capacities; if their problem is clearly identifiable, or they have been referred by someone with a similar complaint and they are prepared to undertake an appropriate course of treatment, and to participate in their own rehabilitation. 'Self-motivational' factors are often crucial to the outcome of anything longer than the briefest clinical interaction. In the case of more stress-related conditions, a preparedness for some difficult self-examination is also very helpful. Where there is chronic pain, such compliance issues may be crucial (Liebenson 1999).

I believe it helps if patients have had to surmount some difficulties in order to get to see the practitioner, for instance:

- a wait for an appointment at a time that may not be easy for them
- some directions to follow if practitioners are off the map of their usual movements
- the effort of organizing their account of the problem
- preparing to be questioned, examined and treated in the first session.

The fact that they are willing to pay for treatment, however small the fee, makes a considerable difference. I have found that, except in longer-term work where budgeting can be difficult, people expect to pay and do not count the cost when their health is at stake.

Timeliness is also crucial. So it helps if patients have understood that the problem is not going to clear up by itself, and they have reached a

---

Box 10.1   Positives: favourable preconditions

- Reputation
- Expectations
- Precise problem
- Self-motivation
- Hurdles
- Self-payment
- Timeliness

point where it simply must be sorted out. All the better then if they have also abandoned previous attempts at treatment with enough time for it to be obvious that these have failed.

These elements can be so powerful that if all are in place it might well matter very little what we as practitioners actually do, provided we fit reasonably well with patients' expectations. In such circumstances I have the strong impression that it is not uncommon for the symptoms to vanish quite suddenly just before the first consultation! Still, we must be sceptical of our own reputation. Consider the case of a patient whom I saw 5 years ago. 'Last time I came in here I was in terrible pain and all bent over. After the first session I walked out straight and completely pain free! You're wonderful; I'm sure you can do that again.' But on checking the case records it seems I struggled for 6 weeks to get the patent out of trouble. Memory gets severely edited!

Beyond the clues we can gather from the bodily responses that we monitor, we just do not know how to assess our efficacy in cases where results come quickly. What I am calling 'placebo' in these examples must actually amount to 'self-cure' and could be interpreted as a form of autosuggestion. In this sort of case I infer that about 80% of the curative effect is due to some spontaneous natural process in the patient. My contribution may have been neutral or may have added or taken away 20%. I think of this patient-produced placebo responsiveness as depending on a favourable momentum (engendered by these positive factors) towards spontaneous or assisted self-cure.

Unfavourable factors

A tendency to a corresponding inertia I would, conversely, ascribe to a number of opposing factors (Box 10.2).

I suspect this opposing set of unfavourable preconditions makes placebo responsiveness and self-cure increasingly unlikely. These include, for instance, if people have just drifted in from the street on the off-chance that they can be seen, or have picked us out of the yellow pages, or if we as

---

Box 10.2 Negatives: unfavourable preconditions

- Unaware of therapist's reputation
- Not self-initiated
- Not paying for self
- Unreasonable expectations
- Unhelpful diagnostic labels
- Current/anticipated compensation claim
- Multiple failures to date
- Multiple current therapists
- No beneficial or adverse effects reported

practitioners are not someone of particular importance to them or to their social contacts. We may seem significantly less important if someone else is footing their bill. Success also comes much harder when patients have been coerced into coming to see us. Moreover success is sometimes impossible when there are legal, occupational, social or medical advantages to be gained from their illness or disability. Unfortunately this 'secondary gain' effect can be at work and may defeat us even when the patient is being consciously entirely honest and honourable.

It is not helpful when patients have unreasonable expectations, nor if they have arrived with unhelpful diagnostic labels. For there is a subtle difference between the person who asks if we can help cure the label (to which they may have grown rather attached) and the person who asks 'please can you help me'? I have found the differences in body language, eye contact and eagerness to interact is usually very marked. And I often notice in retrospect in difficult cases that the initial case history was in fact vague with factors missing, and without the expected clear descriptions and dynamics to the particular symptoms.

The way the illness is labelled can make a huge difference and is subject to the vagaries of medical fashion (Shorter 1992). The intermeshing of labels like 'chronic fatigue syndrome', 'postviral myalgic encephalitis' and 'fibromyalgia syndrome' is always particularly hard to unravel. Discussing this in relation to 'fibromyalgia syndrome' Leon Chaitow, following Hans Selye's ideas about stress and adaptive response, points to a picture of 'allostasis', where homoeostatic processes are so exhausted or poorly formed that even the slightest perturbation is automatically responded to as noxious. This will of course make therapy virtually impossible (Chaitow 2000, p. 27).

A 'cautionary flag' goes up when although patients have seen a succession of other therapists (some of them of good repute and skills) they mention not even a temporary improvement, or if they fail to recount any effort they made themselves on good advice. This flag gets even bigger if they are currently involved with several therapists: a sense of caution amply confirmed when after our initial attempts at treatment the question 'How are you doing?' elicits that same word-for-word vague description of unclear symptoms. We should also beware if at this point we feel challenged to increase our efforts, or feel ineffectual and perhaps even impotent, especially if at the outset we sensed that really the patient did not seem determined to get better. Yet of course a person suffering from long-term chronic pain and disability is likely to be depressed, broke (by the cost of treatment and the loss of work), half-hearted and tempted to grasp at many straws.

Note, however, that these negative predictors could become a self-fulfilling prophecy if they were to undermine and constrain our clinical range. So we need to see them only as broad and generalized indicators, for they may have no relevance to one particular case. It can actually be the most splendid challenge to take on a very difficult, even hopeless-seeming case, and sometimes it is possible to help patients function better and manage their problems with less difficulty despite them.

PERSUASION

Unlike placebo responsiveness, persuasion implies something that the practitioner *does* to the patient. To some extent this is part and parcel of all manual and movement therapies, because necessarily at some point the patient must hand over direction of the session. What use we make of this phenomenon will be crucial to the outcome, especially in brief prognoses. Persuasion can also be very complex (Latey 1984, p. 54):

Under favourable conditions some patients can allow the practitioner almost total influence over their pain sense, proprioceptive sense, pressure sense, location in space, body image, sensations of temperature, and sense of the passage of time itself. We do not know how the patient is induced into the acceptance that our technique is lighter or more painless or less deep or quicker or slower than it really is. There is some sort of useful non-verbal collusion available to us that is unique to physical contact.

Animal hypnosis: a model of non-verbal persuasion for bodyworkers?

Animal magnetism was the 'force' or influence that Anton Mesmer thought he was using in his therapeutic work during the late eighteenth century. The illusion that some magical fluids and esoteric energies are responsible for cure is still with us in spite of all evidence to the contrary. There has been so much study of the effects of persuasion and suggestion (Bowers 1976) that we are bound to examine how this contributes to unorthodox as well as mainstream therapies.

In order to model certain 'persuasive' elements in our physical treatment sessions we might consider the hypnosis of animals. This is largely non-verbal. The production of delusion and illusions through suggestion and manipulation of language though central to hypnosis of the human being is not thought of as an ordinary part of most manual therapies. Its role will be discussed later. But apparently domestic animals and livestock are quite easily hypnotized non-verbally. An excellent method is described by Wilson in 'Dog's hypnosis' (1996). He tells how the owner or trainer can use these techniques to enhance responsiveness and remedy bad habits, as well as for more advanced training. The parallels with bodywork will become clear.

First a special mat or piece of carpet is produced and is only used for the hypnosis sessions, being put away out of sight afterwards. The dog is

---

Box 10.3   Animal hypnosis

- Territory and place
- Restriction of movement
- Direction of movement
- Voice tone
- Repetitions
- Reassurance
- Rewards

---

allowed to play with the mat for a while, then called on to the mat and made to sit or stand. With much reassurance in a soothing voice the dog is told to respond to familiar commands in a relaxed way until accustomed to the trainer. New sorts of behaviour, intended for example to reduce fears or aggression, are introduced calmly and gradually, with return to reassurance and routine whenever the dog seems confused or agitated. The session ends with a couple of familiar movements, an alerting tone of voice and, after rewards are given if it has gone well, the mat is put away.

Within this sequence we can see several features that are common to clinical work (Box 10.3). The time and place are defined as clinical and therapeutic, with the treatment table or exercise mat there, ready to confine the movements and attention of the patient. Special clothing or states of undress further define the interaction. Wilson also makes deliberate use of special smells to mark the hypnotic session for the dog. We all of us know the smell of the hospital, but many other therapy rooms have a distinctive odour. Manual therapy sessions generally begin with cooperation between patients and practitioners. Then the practitioners gradually take over patients' movements, directing them to stand and move in particular ways. Treatment manoeuvres tend to be rhythmical and repetitive, practitioners using steady non-alerting voice tones for their instructions. The end of the session is often marked by encouragement, conveying a sense of achievement, and the return to a more matter-of-fact voice tone reminding patients of helpful advice, homework and the fixing of a next session.

There are many lesser details that can make a difference to the type and intensity of persuasion that we use. We might have a very formal authoritarian type of setting, with white coats, the therapist at a desk, anatomy charts, instruments or machinery; or on the other hand an egalitarian emphasis, with informal clothing, freedom from medical paraphernalia, and identical chairs to sit on. This approach might better suit the more secure practitioner and those patients who approach life with a healthy scepticism. The gender and age of the therapist might also make a difference. But I observe that good therapists seem to be somewhat ageless, and have quite an overlap of traditional gender qualities. Some are also able paradoxically to combine a chameleon-like responsiveness with a very definite sense of self.

Limiting persuasion

When patients hand the direction of the session over they are submitting aspects of themselves for practitioners' use. Therefore as their responsibility lessens so our responsibility must necessarily increase. I think that in fact we do best if we try to minimize our persuasiveness and take great care not to exceed the limits that patients would normally feel comfortable with, both ethically and aesthetically. Even though we are inevitably in charge we must decrease patients' sense of vulnerability and diminish any tendency to dominate. As bodyworkers we should not overwhelm any aspect of them—no matter how much they may seem to want this. In manual therapy we have to capture and engage patients' attention, while at the same time limiting their movement, and taking over direction of their limbs and torso without creating alarm and critical second thoughts. For sustainable work to be useful I also find it is better that patients stay as alert as possible, with the minimum of passivity—for when we are aiming for change across important linked aspects of patients they will need to have all their wits about them if they are to synthesize and integrate much of what is happening in the session. Then, later they will be better able to remember and reflect on interesting aspects of what happened with a clearer mind.

If about 2 minutes into the case history we sense a patient hurrying us to get on with the bodywork, it may be important not to collude. On the table some people want to switch off altogether and become putty in our hands, and to wake up cured after we have done whatever we have to do! It is often difficult then to keep them thinking about their tenseness, and where the tensions are coming from and going to. Talk can be an effective way of keeping them alert and ensuring that most components of their personality stay intact and active. And if both parties are awake then we become gradually more real to one another.

WORKING WITH LONGER PROGNOSES

As so much of our bodywork is quite definitely 'psychosomatic' we are justified in keeping the physical body as the central focus, with the emotions, mind and psychosocial being attended to lightly and tactfully on the periphery. Recognition of this figure–ground relationship is crucial. Yet from time to time this gestalt reverses, providing the interpersonal rapport is good. Then the body may become peripheral to other pressing needs. Often at such times it may be more appropriate for patients just to stay clothed and talk. But that does not mean we should start to think of ourselves as counsellors or psychotherapists. And, very importantly, if we are careful to acknowledge our limitations and learn gradually to expand our capacities then the 'mind' that is allowed to emerge from our bodily understanding might be very different from previous models (see Latey

1996, 1997). This development would not be possible if we had been using more than the minimum of persuasion.

SUGGESTIBILITY

I now want to add to the two original categories of placebo responsiveness and persuasion by drawing two further useful distinctions. These are factors I call 'suggestion' and 'rapport'. Whereas persuasion involves patients just temporarily allowing themselves to do as they are told, suggestion involves a specific attempt to override and alter perceptions and underlying assumptions that patients bring to their inner and outer milieu. Such suggestibility is extremely variable from person to person (Bowers 1976) and may be a measure of the extent to which they can allow external authority to govern their lives and thoughts, and even determine how they feel their own feelings. Suggestibility is essentially passive and uncritical and may have no relation to common sense. Perhaps the tendency to trust, sometimes against our own better reflective judgement, is hardwired: a form of behaviour appropriate to members of a group or herd (Latey 1998). In yielding to group pressure or strong suggestion we are agreeing to agree without being allowed space to question what we are agreeing with. It is as though the perceptions of people who are suggestible can be so easily influenced that at times the only evidence they see is whatever justifies the convictions that they have or that they have been given. And so they lose touch with common sense and healthy questioning far too readily (see, for instance, Chomsky 1989, Gilovich 1991, Livingston 1973, Sargant 1973).

It is clear that strong suggestion applied to suggestible people can have dramatic effects. Dire consequences may, however, follow their 'charismatic' (or sociopathic) use for therapeutic purposes. Consider the case report from a UK colleague in Box 10.4.

Such rapid responses shown in the case study, producing high levels of pain relief, altered perceptions and other strong bodily effects, are not at all unusual because, in the short term at least, the human pain threshold is a highly labile subjective variable. For this reason, hypnotherapists employ numbing of parts of the body as common induction procedures (Calof

---

Box 10.4   Case study

A 50-year-old patient had been working with the osteopath for some months to ease and improve her severely arthritic hip. On impulse she went to a 'faith healer' of grandiose repute. He used strong suggestion to convince her that her hip was pain free and could move fully. She abandoned her stick and walked all the way home in a state of euphoria and religious ecstasy. Next morning she was unable to move from bed. In extreme pain she was taken to hospital and, due to bony collapse, had to have a complete arthrodesis, permanently fusing the joint.

1997). Longer-term effects of strong suggestion are much more variable. My patients who have responded to acupuncture analgesia (administered elsewhere) usually report pain relief that lasts between 2 hours and a week or so. In my experience, lasting results follow only when some underlying problem has also resolved. Unfortunately for patient and practitioner, responses that rely on suggestibility are highly fatigable, and the law of diminishing returns applies. By about the third session the effects of suggestion on the suggestible are exhausted and, though some of these initial effects may be recoverable after a month or so, they never reach the level of the original response.

DEGREE OF DIFFICULTY

In working with difficult problems, we as practitioners get used to estimating severity, complexity and chronicity. We have to gauge the therapeutic time and effort likely to be required and, if we are wise, we judge what I have called the 'momentum' of the patient very carefully (Boxes 10.1 and 2). Then we use only enough persuasion to enable the patients to engage voluntarily in the work; the development of an alliance is a necessary part of any long-term work. Unless we plan to refer them elsewhere, we have to form some ideas about aetiology, prognosis and a treatment programme and agree these with the patient. If we take patients on, the real degree of difficulty will be reflected in the length of the prognosis and the complexity of techniques involved and as the treatment unfolds by whether its aims are actually being met.

More complex work with suggestion (Haley 1973) can be a great help in longer-term manual therapy, particularly when addressing the specific fears, impulses and anxieties that so commonly emerge. Ordinary good humour can be very helpful (Latey 1997). Combinations of suggestion with behavioural modification, guided imagery, narrative development and thought experiment can become quite natural extensions of our ordinary conversations and bodywork. But these techniques require considerable further training, and will need the fully informed consent and cooperation of the patient.

PHASED PATTERNS: THE TRANSITION FROM PERSUASION TO RAPPORT

When working with long-term complex problems I have found that a familiar pattern tends to occur (Box 10.5). If complex patients have, say, five predominant aspects to their complaint they might start with a quite dramatic improvement in as many as four of these during the opening phase. The fifth may remain stubbornly present throughout these early sessions.

Box 10.5 Phased patterns in long-term treatment

1. **Opening stage (and brief cases)**
   - Importance of 'patient momentum'
   - Patient responsiveness and autosuggestion
   - Practitioner persuasion/specific suggestion (minimal in complex cases)

2. **Refractory phase**
   - Patient unresponsive
   - Gradual return of symptoms
   - Gains lost
   - Practitioner frustrated; quick-fix measures fail

3. **Developing rapport**
   - Good working relationship
   - Confidence in effectiveness: focused effort is worthwhile
   - Some integration, sense of control and meaning

4. **Phases of recurrence**
   - Longest phase
   - Confidence is strained
   - Same areas recycle for second and third time

5. **Quiescence**
   - Calming down, increasingly symptom free for longer
   - Questing around for new work

6. **Discharge and follow-up**
   - Patient unsure if ready to disengage
   - Practitioner retreats to more 'distance'
   - Need for reassurance and suggestion

In the next phase very little seems to happen to the symptoms themselves, but the patient and therapist adjust to each other and find new ways of relating. Gradually the symptoms return, perhaps during a trial of 'no treatment'.

In the third phase each area of complaint will tend in turn to move into prominence as different bodily regions, functions and subject matter become the focus of the work. This third phase is very satisfying if symptoms, bodily work and other concerns begin to make sense. Even then, though some sort of integration seems to be happening, the main symptoms generally do not disappear altogether.

At least two periods of relapse and reworking usually follow. To me this fourth phase, by far the longest, feels as if the body were refusing to change its position till the third time around. And I nearly always have to keep emphasizing with the patient how healthy an idiosyncratic streak of extreme stubbornness can be because we have to respect that intimate core of individuality and let it remain entirely intact and unchallenged. This fourth stage is a major challenge for us as practitioners, who have to be very patient, surmounting our own frustration and boredom while remaining alert for missing elements, avoiding repetition and inventing fresh ways of covering the same ground.

In the fifth phase there is a combination of quiescence and complacency alongside a searching around for more work to do. For, as sessions are spaced further apart, the symptom-free periods lengthen to the point where symptoms are hardly mentioned, though they may recur in a minor form just before each session. These are clear signs that the therapeutic process is coming to an end and the patient and practitioner will now have to prepare to disengage.

In the sixth and final phase, the ending of the work, there is often a brief return to the need for reassurance. I nearly always feel it helpful to offer continuing support if it is needed from time to time, observe that I will miss the patient I have got to know so well and generally set the scene for follow-up.

The effects of the patient's momentum, the persuasiveness of the therapist and the setting, as well as any initial suggestions that have been used, are usually exhausted by the end of the second phase. From the third phase onwards it is the clinical framework and setting, the rapport and the joint efforts of practitioner and patient that do the work. Only in the ending might we have to return to a more stylized and formal way of working.

INTERPERSONAL AND 'PHYSICAL' RAPPORT

In interactions where there is no need for a durable rapport there will always be an imbalance between activity and passivity, dominance and submissiveness. Unclear boundaries of various other sorts are likely to be significant (and potentially hazardous to both patient and practitioner) too. But in phase three of the therapeutic pattern (Box 10.5) both participants are present in a more equal way. Control and direction of the interaction is now passing back and forth. It would not be surprising then if the clinical skills most relevant to tackling chronic and difficult problems depended more on interpersonal rapport than used to be thought. There is evidence that this is so for patients in psychotherapy, the only field where long-term clinical work has been studied. It seems that good results, in that field at least, have far more to do with the quality of rapport than with practitioners' espoused theories or training schools (Roth & Fonagy 1996). There are even some aspects of psychotherapy where the 'untrained' (and by implication the most naturally 'en rapport') may do best of all (Spinelli 1999).

In my experience, the unfolding of a longer-term clinical relationship is marked by the way questions, ideas, pauses, wry comments and tentative answers increase and flow freely—with lots of requests aimed at expansion of each other's viewpoint in interesting areas. My job then is partly to keep steady progress, with the ability to introduce refreshing differences, and partly to maintain an exquisite sensitivity to what I call 'flinch'. As body-workers we must carefully monitor the impressions we are making, and the responses evoked. Sensitivity to this 'flinch' boundary is not only critical to the work of physical contact but is also a part of sustaining an interpersonal rapport through conversation and listening.

In physical work if we have good 'tissue empathy' we are used to monitoring the responses of tissue tone and muscles, as follows:

- Is the patient able to relax with what we are doing without dissociating?
- Do the patient's muscles contract back against us?
- Do we notice a slight catch in the patient's breathing?
- Are the patient's hands or feet curling?
- Is there a slight flicker or grimace at the side of the patient's face?
- Are we checking how sore the patient feels in areas we are working on?

In conversation with patients we can also be watching for parallel signs of recoil:

- Have they suddenly gone very silent for a moment?
- Did they suddenly withdraw for an instant, and freeze their smile?
- Do we know when we have overstepped the mark, and must change tack and offer prompt apology?

In the 1880s A. T. Still was bringing osteopathy together from his work as a bonesetter and magnetic healer. At the same time Sigmund Freud was himself using hypnosis, massage and head pressure while he discussed with the patient what memories and images came to mind. There was much interest in therapeutic suggestion at that time (e.g. Bernheim 1888). Sadly, just as psychoanalysis retreated from physical rapport, so too did osteopathy retreat from psychological awareness—to the great loss of both professions.

When closely engaged with a patient's body, the practitioner will inevitably be touched and moved. It seems to me that this 'attunement' with the patient's inner movement involves more than just the proprioceptive and locomotor senses of our muscularity. Though in themselves these perceptions constitute a largely ignored 'sixth sensory system' we may in addition be interacting in three other ways. These entail an interaction between our emotional, visceral and 'mental' patterns of muscular sensation: the embodied awareness of movement and being that constitute the lived experience of each person in all of its layered complexity (Latey 1979, 1996). In a very real way we can sense a great deal about one another.

PRACTITIONERS AND THEIR FEELINGS

Normally this semiconscious bodily and emotional exchange proceeds unremarkably. But sometimes there can be unpredictable reactions between patients and their manual therapists. Because we have poor differentiation of these senses, and even less language for them, these experiences tend to be 'synaesthetic'. They can induce strong echoes in senses that are otherwise disengaged. In my own work this can mean feeling deeply moved sometimes, as if swirled slowly in a tidal undercurrent in the sea, or as if caught in powerful magnetic fields. Other practitioners have described experiencing colours, vibrations and resonant shapes that are not there, or more rarely sounds, tastes and smells. In conversation with colleagues, feelings of fluidity, 'melting' and drifting are the most common. In my opinion this may explain why people have needed to invent esoteric energies and magical auras to account for mysterious aspects of the therapeutic relationship. Perhaps a better understanding of the mutual rhythm of our therapeutic 'dance' with the patient would also reduce the confusion surrounding the involuntary movement patterns we are so familiar with as bodyworkers, and help us understand their clinical significance (Latey 1979, 1985).

Structural coupling and intertransference

Chilean biologist-philosophers Humberto Maturana & Francisco Varela (1980) make a useful set of distinctions about interactions between objects, cells and organisms. These concepts immediately impressed me and I think they add to our understanding of clinical rapport and particularly of physical rapport in bodywork. These authors distinguish two kinds of interaction. The first, which they call 'instructive interaction' occurs when two objects interact in an exact and predictable way. Maturana & Varela point out that living organisms never respond to perturbation in this way because their response is always determined by their own particular developmental history, which itself depends on an idiosyncratic self-structuring they call 'autopoiesis' (Maturana & Varela 1980). Instead, when two living organisms are in close interaction, a process of mutual recursive change (named 'structural coupling') is initiated. According to Maturana & Varela, multicellular organisms could not have evolved without some such sharing of one another's restructuring processes. The mutual 'tuning in' that such an evolutionary leap requires they term 'second-order autopoiesis'. But they do not envisage this as the kind of direct mechanical coupling we see in a gear train or study in spinal biomechanics; it is closer to the phenomenon of 'entrainment' (e.g. resonance between identical tuning forks) and relates to the notion of 'emergence' that features in the idea of complexity in chaos theory (Davies 1989).

Between 'social' organisms structural coupling would seem to be both more intermittent and less intense. But the possibility that it exists has obvious consequences for any interpretation of human interactions, especially in therapeutic work and particularly in bodywork. For here we are faced with the difference between trying to *make* change happen and tuning in to engage in such a way as to *allow* changes to happen. This is a highly significant distinction—the more so when we recognize that structural coupling cannot possibly be unidirectional and that our own personal plasticity and mutability are therefore an essential element in something we could call 'clinical structural coupling'. These notions do not fit well though with dualistic views of persuasion, suggestion and placebo responsiveness and they clearly subvert a purely mechanical view of manual therapies. What is happening here is different and it is happening to both parties, though they will perceive it differently. The author has previously named the phenomenon 'intertransference' (Latey 1979, p. 105).

Intimacy in the therapeutic relationship

Even though it might seem completely beyond the scope of the non-touching psychotherapist's models, in fact a great deal has been written about the exchange of mental contents and bodily sensations in the psychotherapeutic relationship, and most notably about its dangers. However, I consider that psychotherapists' fear of regression, fragmentation and sexual abuse may be all the more pertinent because their work lacks a bodily anchor. In the process of bodywork there are undeniable parallels with sexual coupling: two people alone in a warm room, with undressing, fleshy contact and handling of parts. Yet although this physically close relationship can make clinical structural coupling more likely I believe it is unlikely to happen at all unless the relationship is *participative*.

But the sexual metaphor also extends into other approaches: we could say that the hypnotherapist is metaphorically seducing compliance, or that the faith healer in the previous example overpowered the woman and in doing so ravaged the integrity of her pelvic structure. In benign contrast, any meeting of minds can be a sort of 'mating' wherein lies the potential for generating new ideas about living; wherever clinical structural coupling works well we could say there has been 'therapeutic conception and gestation': new life gained for the patient. I am in no doubt that manual therapy, in the terms related in this chapter, can from time to time bring about such a subtle coming together of renewed patients: with boundaries intact, softer and more resilient where they had been brittle, healing where they were wounded or ill formed, and more distinct where they had been blurred. Lesser degrees of clinical structural coupling are probably an ordinary everyday part of good manual therapy practice, just as they are an important aspect of the empathy we bring to our daily work and relationships.

An intimacy of adults that is neither sexual nor infantile is possible and, I think, a vitally important part of life and health. As an example, I ask you to imagine a widow and a widower who have known each other for years. Though they are not a couple, at a reunion party they dance together and, in the last slow waltz, we watch them as they become very close, leaning in to each other. Dancing, their swaying movement is no longer in time to the music, but slowly it wanders chaotically around a small area of the floor. Looking at them you sense a deep warmth of shared affection, sadness, happiness, compassion and contentment. A few minutes later they have parted, leaving for their separate homes, perhaps hoping they might meet again next year, feeling some healthy tiredness and a little heartache. Yet something has unfrozen for them: they can breathe more easily even if just to sigh.

CONCLUSION

To some degree all of our successes as manual therapists could be ascribed to the working, in one form or another, of placebo response and persuasion. It is up to us to determine which form. I have tried here to begin by distinguishing between the rapid results of brief procedures and the complex pattern of phases that we meet in longer-term work. Though many effects of touch and movement have not been mentioned in this paper (see, for example, Nathan 1999), it appears to the author that touch can for some people be a way of restoring 'felt identity'. In its capacity to bring this about, I have implied a contrast between the outcome of effective manual therapy and the potential for unreality and instability entailed in non-touch methods. I do so because in my experience touch can defuse excesses of transference and countertransference (see Ch. 8). None the less touch, because it is so sorely needed in our alienated society, can on its own also be deeply addictive; tangible separation can be an emotional loss for both parties. So there are clearly many dangers and contraindications not discussed in this chapter that are inherent in this approach to manual therapy. There is all the more reason then to distinguish between persuasion, suggestion, patients' momentum and their suggestibility, and to be extremely curious about treatment rapport, especially in difficult cases.

The author's *Muscular Manifesto* (Latey 1979) started from the premise that when the problem can be viewed simply then impressive and satisfying 'cures' can come from 'a palpable consensual condensation' between osteopath and patient. But the depth of understanding, compassion and skill to enable this to work with complicated patients dawns slowly in today's hurried society. With difficult patients I am accustomed to waiting hopefully, with considerable optimism about our human capacity for self-righting.

REFERENCES

Bernheim H 1888 Suggestive therapeutics: a treatise on the nature and uses of hypnotism. Putnams, New York
Bowers K 1976 Hypnosis for the seriously curious. Norton, New York

Calof D 1997 The couple who became each other. Century, London

Chaitow L 2000 Fibromyalgia syndrome. Churchill Livingstone, New York, p 27

Chomsky N 1989 Necessary illusions; thought control in democratic societies. CBC, Montreal, Canada

Davies P 1989 The cosmic blueprint. Unwin, London, pp 149, 150

Gilovich T 1991 How we know what isn't so. The fallibility of reason in everyday life. Free Press/Macmillan, New York

Haley J 1973 Uncommon therapy. Norton, New York

Latey P 1979 The muscular manifesto, 2nd edn. Osteopathic Publishing, London

Latey P 1984 An expansion of osteopathic theory of technique. British Osteopathic Journal 19:51–56

Latey P 1985 Cranial osteopathy: a divisive alternative. Journal of Alternative Medicine 3(10):6, 7

Latey P 1996 Feelings, muscles and movement. Journal of Bodywork and Movement Therapies 1(1):44–52

Latey P 1997 Complexity and the changing individual. Journal of Bodywork and Movement Therapies 1(5):270–279

Latey P 1998 The pressures of the group. Journal of Bodywork and Movement Therapies 2(2):115–124

Liebenson C 1999 Motivating pain patients to become more active. Journal of Bodywork and Movement Therapies 3:143–146

Livingston A 1973 Dealing with cheats. Lippincott, Philadelphia

Maturana H, Varela F 1980 Autopoiesis and cognition. Riedel, Holland

Nathan B 1999 Touch and emotion in manual therapy. Churchill Livingstone, New York

Roth A, Fonagy P 1996 What works for whom: a critical review of psychotherapy research. Guilford, New York

Sargant W 1973 The mind possessed. A physiology of possession, mysticism and faith healing. Heinemann, Oxford

Shorter E 1992 From paralysis to fatigue—a history of psychosomatic illness in the modern era. Free Press/Macmillan, New York

Spinelli E 1999 If there are so many psychotherapies how come we keep making the same mistakes? Psychotherapy in Australia 6(1):19

Wilson S F T 1996 Dog's hypnosis. BluePrint, Bankstown, Sydney

---

FURTHER READING

For studies of synaesthesia in other fields the following is recommended:

Baron-Cohen S, Harrison J E (eds) 1997 Synaesthesia. Blackwell, Oxford

10

Healing and Therapeutic Touch: is it all in the mind?

Stephen G. Wright and Jean Sayre-Adams

What is Therapeutic Touch?	A TT case study
Intention in TT	Placebos, energies, fields and consciousness
Two models of TT	
Stages of TT	Conclusion: we are all in this together

Editor's note

Several practitioners have told us how they think the 'practitioner effect' works. Anton de Craen's chapter (Ch 12) suggests that just conveying an optimistic prediction about the outcome of treatment is not enough. So there have to be more to the practitioner effect than this: *intention* apparently plays a part and the practitioner's authentic expectation that his intention could actually in some way change the person being treated. It is easier to understand how this conviction is conveyed by an actual prescription, or by touch, as they are something concrete. Successful psychotherapy uses language in a way that Angela Clow tells us may translate into nerve activity and trigger a cascade of brain-related neuro-hormonal release pervading the organism. Yet the mere verbal attempt to promote positive expectation is, according to de Craen, not enough. So although language (verbal and non-verbal, conscious and unconscious) is clearly part and parcel of the effect, perhaps in order be effective it must convey authenticity, conviction, intention and relatedness. It seems to me that these aspects weave through and connect together what our authors' had written about the effect. But in the case of a category of treatments we might call 'healing' these aspects are the totality of the therapy; all other elements having been stripped away, the therapy itself is entirely non-specific. It it only works when a practitioner believes it works, then how does the client know they believe it? I asked two leading exponents for their ideas about intention and how the ability to communicate that intention might depend on their belief about is impact.

If you don't know what to do,
Just put your hands on them and love them.

Pannatier

When words fail, there may be no other way of communicating to a patient that 'I care' than by touch. However, there are many ways of touching and even more ways in which the patient might respond. With burgeoning interest in access to the complementary therapies (Woodham & Peters 1997), and after considerable initial hostility from the 'orthodox' professionals, a steady increase in emphasis on acceptance and integration with mainstream healthcare (Featherstone & Forsyth 1997, Foundation for Integrated Medicine 1997) has stimulated deeper awareness of the possibilities for healing.

A view of two distinct models has emerged as a result. Orthodox medicine is seen as essentially reductionist, concerning itself primarily with identifying a disease and intervening with an appropriate treatment. Complementary medicine is regarded as holistic, having as its primary concern an attempt to see the patient as a whole person and promote the mobilization of the patient's own healing resources.

These views are themselves reductionist, belying the immense intricacy and complexity of healing. Not all orthodox practitioners are unquestioningly committed to the traditional medical model of diagnosis, disease and treatment. Nor is the rhetoric of holism always matched by the reality of complementary therapy practice. It is equally possible to hear reports from patients of doctors and nurses working holistically in traditional healthcare settings (Taylor 1994) as it is to hear of complementary therapists who limit their healing potential by their overattachment to the technical aspects of their therapy (Wright & Sayre-Adams 1999).

This chapter takes up the example of one technique, Therapeutic Touch (TT). Widely adopted by healthcare professionals, especially nurses, it now forms part of accredited programmes of education in many schools of medicine and nursing (Sayre-Adams & Wright 1995). Like many other therapies, it has provoked diverse responses among mainstream practitioners. In some settings it has been uncritically accepted; others have rigorously researched it. Despite such studies TT often meets with deep scepticism, although elsewhere it is enthusiastically applied. And, even though standards have been set for its use in conventional units, in the minds of many who see it at work the question remains: is TT an effective treatment, or is it simply a placebo response whose benefit largely depends on the 'recipient' believing in it? The observation that research into the placebo response demonstrates that it is none the less a response (whereby the patient's health status actually changes not only subjectively but also according to objective physiological measures) only makes the question more complex: after all, TT also has a considerable body of good quality research attesting to its effectiveness in these same terms. Even so, many of these studies, perhaps in order to gain acceptance within the orthodox paradigm, focus on the use of TT as though it were a type of 'health technology' practised by someone upon someone else. This frames the practice of TT in terms of the classic conventional medical model: identify and name the problem, then do something to the patient in order to resolve it. This perspective creates substantial problems for understanding TT. In fact the TT model itself implies that whether one is aiming to practise holistically or just seeking to understand the healing milieu then a more comprehensive model is called for. First because the diagnosis–intervention–outcome model ignores the participation of the patient. Second because TT aims to take account of the total, essentially unified, context in which healing processes emerge. And thirdly because putting this theory into practice requires TT practitioners to use their understanding, imagination and consciousness in particular ways.

WHAT IS THERAPEUTIC TOUCH?

A detailed exploration of TT is beyond the scope of this chapter. Briefly, it can be seen as a modern version of one of the oldest of therapies: the use of touch as a means of comfort and healing. The term 'Therapeutic Touch' was coined by Dr Dolores Krieger, professor of nursing at New York University, working with Dora Kunz, then President of the American Theosophical Society, who laid the foundations for the practice and research of TT in the early 1970s.

Capital letters are used for Therapeutic Touch to distinguish it from other forms of therapeutic touch such as laying on of hands, massage, stroking, hand holding and so on. Touch is a core element in nursing. The distinct forms and processes of TT that have entered mainstream healthcare education, particularly among nurses, are well documented (e.g. Krieger 1979, Sayre-Adams & Wright 1995). (For further information on TT, see the address at the end of this text.)

Intention in TT

TT is viewed as a natural human potential that can be learned and practised by anyone who has an *intention* to help or heal. This intention is at the core of the TT process and involves an attempt to focus on the well-being of the patient in an act of unconditional love and compassion (Quinn 1993). For this reason Krieger called it 'a healing meditation' (Krieger, Peper & Ancoli 1979).

Two models of TT

Krieger initially explained TT in terms of the vedic notions of prana and chakras (Krieger 1979). Krieger's early idea was similar to the theoretical underpinnings of Reiki and spiritual healing. She conceived of healing 'energy' moving from one person or other source to the other person needing healing.

TT has more recently been linked to Martha Rogers' 'science of unitary human beings' (Rogers 1990, Sayre-Adams & Wright 1995), a particular nursing theory that is allied to modern systems thinking as represented in, for example, holism, chaos theory and quantum physics (Bohm 1973, Dossey 1997, Zohar 1990). Rogers presents a nursing theory that considers human beings as integrated wholes interacting with a universe where each part influences every other. Indeed, in an intensely holistic model such as this, the word 'part' is itself an oxymoron: a term used only to convey the concept that we ourselves and the universe are not a series of parts, but a vast unified pattern of which our limited senses discern only a limited picture.

In this view TT is a participatory process. Rogers' model offers a different perspective from that of Krieger: a mutual process of all the involved patterns. Healing emerges as all involved participate consciously in the healing environment. The important difference is that, whereas the former may be seen as a *directive*, even a unidirectional process, from healer to patient, the latter is not directional and simply entails a conscious *awareness* of the healing environment and an intention to heal.

With no focus on specific outcomes or intervening technique, the essence of TT is that to 'work' there must be no expectation of an outcome. If there is a goal at all, it is to make the person whole, with no fixed agenda of what wholeness might be for the other person. The use of the hands and other practices in TT are simply ways to shift awareness and consciousness. They are only an outward expression of what is happening, an immeasurable but conscious participation in the 'sacred space' (Wright & Sayre-Adams 2000), where healing emerges from the right relationship. This relationship is not just between healer and patient, but with the whole environmental field. It is a mutual process, where even words like 'healer' and 'patient' and 'environmental field' are themselves problematic. Because they separate and reduce, these terms fail to convey the essential participatory immersion. In the safe, sacred space for healing everything is interconnected: 'patient', 'healer', 'environment' do not stand apart. At an 'energetic' level there is a merging, a union, that is not a collation of identities. 'Healer' and 'patient' thus participate in a healing process where both are affected.

Stages of TT

In the process of TT, four stages or phases are generally distinguished. Once again we have to fracture the process in order to describe it. But, bearing this in mind, the four phases can be described as the following.

• **Centring**. By shifting awareness from an external to an internal focus, the practitioner becomes relaxed and calm and makes a mental intention to be available for healing the patient. Being 'centred' the practitioner may enter what is described as a meditative state of 'being in the here and now'. Undistracted and focused on the moment, the practitioner is at the same time in a state of alertness as attention is brought especially to the hands and fully engaged with the patient and the healing process.

• **Assessment**. The practitioner's hands are passed over the patient's body, noticing areas of difference: any sensations of heat, cold, heaviness, tingling. Any intuitive insight or sense of knowing about what is going on with the patient is noted. These and other qualities may be recognized as the healer seeks to get a sense of the patient's 'energy field'.

• **Clearing**. The hands are used to shape a symmetrical and rhythmical 'flow of energy' throughout the field. This entails sweeping the hands above and along the length of the patient's body, paying particular attention to any area to which awareness was drawn during the assessment.

• **Repatterning**. The practitioner returns to the places where these imbalances were noticed in the assessment and focuses on a repatterning of the 'field' through intention and imagery. (Note that healers should also be aware of their own 'field' and how this is simultaneously a part of the patient's 'field'.)

A TT CASE STUDY

In the vignette in Box 11.1 (from Sayre-Adams & Wright 1995) we see these categories reflected in a TT practitioner's case study. Although the above phases have been distinguished, the vignette illustrates how the process of TT is more an interactive flow than a series of linear 'action–reaction' events.

This short case study illustrates some of the main elements of TT. Perhaps it also helps us understand why, like many complementary therapies, it has often had a difficult, if not hostile, reception in conventional settings. The process is entirely subjective. Both parties rely on their own lived experience and the practitioner monitors and evaluates the effects qualitatively. And there is little that could be called objective about this typical report. Neither can one point to rational, scientific and observable actions and outcomes, though changes in patients' appearance and function as well as their own reports of changing would clearly be significant here. Moreover, in the case detailed there are many possible variables affecting Mr J.'s well-being. So it is impossible for an outside assessor to ascribe Mr J.'s reported benefit directly to TT itself. Furthermore the whole encounter, though structured around a certain state of consciousness and shaped by the procedures defined by TT practice, could equally well be attributed to a multitude of independent and unpredictable variables. The practitioner speaks of 'energy' and 'fields', and makes reference to intuition and altered states of awareness: hardly the language of mainstream practice. The practitioner also seeks quite overtly to establish a type

---

Box 11.1 Case study

Mr J. was a 61-year-old farmer with very unsteady gait. Because of this he had many falls and minor injuries and was often mistaken as being drunk. He told me his problem was due to a hereditary disease for which his own doctor had told him that nothing could be done.

Before starting TT, I centred myself, visualizing an oak tree with its leaves shimmering in a gentle breeze. Inwardly calming myself, I took a series of deep breaths, and just imagined myself as being very present with this patient, letting all other thoughts drift away. I paid attention to my hands, felt them relaxed and ready to receive whatever I was to notice.

With Mr J. lying down, I began the initial assessment. I had an overall sense of coolness in his energy field. As I had not felt any particular block or other differences, my intuition led me gently to move towards his abdominal area and begin the repatterning. So I imagined a warm, soothing light encompassing him. I again moved my hands in a head to toe direction to reassess and continued the repatterning, moving my hands in a continuous, flowing manner. I kept this up for about 10 minutes, until a feeling of warmth replaced the previous coolness. When I then worked on his back, I felt the same feeling of coolness down the spinal column. After the repatterning this too was replaced by warmth. Mr J. told me he had no obvious sensations, but said that 'inwardly something has happened' and asked 'is it possible to feel better immediately?' His gait was unchanged.

The following week he returned 'over the moon' about how he felt. He called me the 'lady with the oilcan'. He said his joints were no longer stiff and that he had not fallen all week. He was now able to manage the steps in his house without having to hold on to the doorframe and told me he could put his shoes on without having to sit down.

On the second and third visits I found there were still areas of coolness in the energy fields around his legs and spinal column. I experienced shocks like static discharges. When a repatterning was done at the third visit Mr J. told me he had felt 'a sensation travelling down my body'.

Three weeks later he had his fourth and final session. At this time his energy field felt complete and he had not fallen for 6 weeks. His unsteady gait was still evident, but less exaggerated and he felt better able to get about.

---

of connection and involvement with the client that orthodox medicine would probably find objectionable. For this is not the account of an aloof health carer at work, but rather someone who is *intimately* involved with her own and (she would claim) her patient's processes. What is more, the claim that practice is grounded in what is considered as literally *intersubjective* experience (see Ch. 9) would seem to many conventional healthcare workers to be positively parapsychological, and therefore highly suspect. How could such sharing possibly occur? For those of a sceptical persuasion all these issues are grist to their mill. Of course, many of the same issues apply across the range of complementary therapies, and naturally they provoke similar objections.

On these grounds, 'orthodoxy' summarily rejects the many positive case histories about TT and the numerous research studies published. If any effect is acknowledged at all, it is to dismiss claims by patients and practitioners as 'mere placebo response'. Yet evidence for the effects of TT on wound healing, anxiety, the promotion of relaxation or altered perceptions of pain and the provision of comfort in the dying process is strong

(Richardson 1995). The problem of replicating these studies has fuelled this scepticism even in those cases where the scientifically acceptable methodology of the double-blind, randomized, controlled trial has been employed. For instance, if a patient's *feeling* of well-being after therapy has been used as an outcome measure then this is likely to be dismissed as a placebo response, even if discernible physiological changes have also taken place.

PLACEBOS, ENERGIES, FIELDS AND CONSCIOUSNESS

One definition of placebo is 'any procedure that produces an effect in a patient because of its therapeutic intent and not its specific nature', and other chapters in this text (see Section 1) have dealt with this issue in more detail. In relation to TT, this is a paradoxical definition since the intent is itself considered to be specific and the outcome of TT is conceived of as being due to a repatterning of the subject's 'energy field', in order that self-healing can occur. TT practitioners believe that all healing is necessarily self-healing. More interdisciplinary research is required to validate what is actually taking place, and to explore the whole nature of what have been named as 'energy fields'.

The notion of fields and energy are frequently evoked in so-called 'New Age' settings. Cutting-edge thinkers in the fields of consciousness research and quantum physics use the same terms, which perhaps suggests there could be an authentically 'energetic' basis for therapies such as TT. TT is couched in the language of modern science but its theories clearly resonate with ancient ideas of a universal energy that forms itself into fields. Something like this can be found in many different cultures: the Chinese refer to 'qi', the Indians to 'prana' and amongst the Jews it is 'ruach'. TT practitioners believe they are working with this same 'energy' and that it puts the person into the best state for self-healing to occur. Modern science recognizes only four forms of energy: gravity, strong and weak nuclear forces and the energies in the electromagnetic spectrum. 'New Age' jargon uses the word 'energy' liberally, yet offers no clear definition of what is meant nor how it does what it does. Although it may be that there are other 'subtle energies' at work, as the proponents of TT claim and on which Rogers bases her theory, such claims need to be made with caution. It is not just that their existence is difficult to substantiate; for despite the quantum parallels the 'New Age' loves to draw this 'life energy' is strictly *not* one of science's four forces. So, postulating its existence as the a priori basis of TT exposes the technique to ridicule and makes it almost impossible to advance our understanding of these approaches in the scientific community.

None the less, it should be apparent that there are aspects of consciousness that lie outside the common realm just as there are spectra of energy far beyond what our five senses are capable of perceiving. Pribram (1991) believes our brains have learned to edit our ordinary reality, and that this editing function could include the capacity to see or feel, for instance, human energy fields. Until recently the texts describing and exploring these ideas stood entirely outside the conventional mainstream. Yet it may be relevant that in our postmodern times what is being revealed at the leading edge of physics and consciousness studies seems to bear little resemblance to the world we recognize with our five senses.

Dossey (1997) believes that it may be justifiable to use the term 'energy' only in a provisional, qualified, metaphorical way. To do otherwise, apart from exposing the idea to ridicule, may be to limit or blind us to the true nature of healing. There is no denying that in the practice of TT many people experience something unusual; whether it is 'energy' or not is open to question. Until understanding of the concept deepens or further research links these experiences with more objective, measurable and concrete outcomes, the term ought to be used only metaphorically. Likewise, notions of 'consciousness' are changing. The term no longer implies only the part of the mind that is aware, but embraces both the conscious and unconscious self. The jungian view of the unconscious sees it as the seat of timeless psychic forces. From Newman's (1986) perspective health is a state of constantly expanding consciousness. In holistic terms, consciousness far from being the by-product of functioning neurons becomes the very stuff that binds the universe together. From these perspectives we *are* consciousness, we are in consciousness and consciousness is in us.

Pert's (1997) cutting-edge work in psychoneuroimmunology lends scientific credence to a current style of thinking that intertwines the nature of consciousness, energy and holism. For example, her research work and writing demonstrate an extraordinary interconnectedness between emotions and physiological effects on the body. In her view, mind, body, emotions and spirit, hitherto often discussed as distinct entities, are part of an interconnected whole person. In turn the whole person is embedded in all of creation, and she insists that the emotions form the unifying thread between all of them. Her theory of multilevelled interconnectedness reminds us how primitive our understanding of healing has hitherto been, and that how we work with healing is intimately bound up with our conscious participation in it.

CONCLUSION: WE ARE ALL IN THIS TOGETHER

If we are patterns of 'energy' (however we perceive these to be) resonating with one other, then 'each' and 'other' begin to lose their usual meaning. As John Heron so clearly explains in Chapter 13, given that this is the case the nature of healing enters a new paradigm. The traditional, reductionist 'I do this to you' approach is no longer explanatory when we are not separate. And, though this participatory world view paints a radically different picture of reality, it is not one divorced from mainstream discourse of science, philosophy and practice, as Heron explains. Here is an important new (yet also ancient) metaphor that seems to resonate at a personal level with metaphors used in neuroscience, holography, systems theory and particle physics. The consequences for our understanding of healing processes are far reaching, not least because by intentionally, consciously, seeking the healing of another we would heal ourselves: the mutuality involved means that the practitioner of TT is affected by this process as well. It is not unidirectional from 'healer' to 'patient'. McClelland's (1985) study, for example, suggests that when people feel unconditional love or compassion (an essential part of the TT process) this feeling may have an added benefit by enhancing the immune processes of the practitioner too. This raises the possibility of conducting research to confirm the many reports of TT practitioners who claim they feel better after working with patients. Is TT practice truly associated with less likelihood of sickness and lower absenteeism from work (Sayre-Adams & Wright 1995)?

We have tried to suggest so far that TT can be interpreted as giving clues about previously unsuspected intersubjective influences on healing outcomes, and that therefore it hints at processes having an important bearing on what has been wrongly dismissed as 'mere placebo effects'. TT may be viewed as a simple technique, based on some as yet unsubstantiated claims about healing energy, whereby one person does something to another. Viewed through that lens, TT emerges, albeit with a dubious theoretical base, much the same as any other spanner for the health engineer. Of course, if TT is simply a technique then it can be learned and practised like any other, with one person tapping into some as yet mysterious energy source to heal another.

We prefer to understand TT as a medium for 'being with' rather than for 'doing to' another person. Having shifted TT from being simply a technique we have looked at some of the implications: that TT aims through intention to make the practitioner available to the other, that to do this it relies on a particular state of consciousness and the participatory nature of reality, and that it aims to put the patient in the best condition for nature to act. Florence Nightingale wrote in 1869 that this is the purpose of nursing. As Reilly points out in Chapter 7, we can bracket the impact of this style of 'being with' as 'placebo response', but the term tends to confuse because it obscures a valuable and potentially transformative reorientation of the practitioner–client axis. So, is this the action of 'placebo response', 'triggered' by the 'loving, trusting presence' of another in the 'therapeutic relationship'? Perhaps, but this description rushes past a series of significant factors (we have put them in quotes) that apparently determine such a highly desirable outcome. There are many ways of depicting this process. But we have found that the language and models enshrined in TT can facilitate these factors and allow the learning and attitudes required for effective practice. They entail a shift in consciousness (known as 'centre-ing') a focusing on interconnectedness (through an 'energy field'), and an intention to allow the being (physiological, mental–emotional, spiritual) of the other person to re-cognize or re-member a lost, but inherent, healthy mode.

Our experience as practitioners working with TT who have taught it to thousands of nurses and other healthcare workers supports an impression that seems central to this reorientation. Reilly's chapter also bears it out: that our willingness to be with patients in this way may be part of our own inner pathway towards wholeness. This desire to be whole, to heal (and both words have their origins in the same teutonic root word *'haelan'* meaning whole, hale, healthy, at one with oneself) seems to be an inherent drive in each of us.

Mark Young (1995), an osteopath and Sufi, has noted: 'There can be a moment in healing when there is perfect balance and all distinction between healer and wounded disappears. At this point something else can enter and both can be transported to a place of mystery. Part of us yearns to return to this place, because it is here that we are made whole.'

REFERENCES

Bohm D 1973 Quantum theory as an indication of a new order in physics: implicit and explicit order in physical law. Foundation of Physics 3: 139–168
Dossey L 1997 The forces of healing: reflections on energy, consciousness and the beef stroganoff principle. Alternative Therapies 3(5):8–13
Featherstone C, Forsyth L 1997 Medical marriage: the new partnership between orthodox and complementary medicine. Findhorn Press, Findhorn
Foundation for Integrated Medicine 1997 Integrated healthcare: a way forward for the next five years? FIM, London
Krieger D 1979 The therapeutic touch: how to use your hands to help or heal. Prentice Hall, New York
Krieger D, Peper E, Ancoli S 1979 Physiologic indices of therapeutic touch. American Journal of Nursing 14:660–662
McClelland M 1985 Cited in Quinn J 1993 Psychoimmunologic effects of therapeutic touch on practitioners and recently bereaved recipients: a pilot study. Advanced Nursing Science 15(4):13–26
Newman M 1986 Health as expanding consciousness. C V Mosby, St Louis, MO
Nightingale F 1869 (reprint 1980) Notes on nursing: what it is and what it is not. Churchill Livingstone, New York
Pert C 1997 Molecules of emotion. Scribner, New York
Pribram K 1991 Cited in Talbot M 1991 The holographic universe. HarperCollins, New York
Quinn J 1993 Psychoimmunologic effects of therapeutic touch on practitioners and recently bereaved recipients: a pilot study. Advanced Nursing Science 15(4):13–26
Richardson M 1995 A review of the literature and research. In: Sayre-Adams J, Wright S G (eds) The theory and practice of therapeutic touch. Churchill Livingstone, New York
Rogers M 1990 Nursing; science of unitary, irreducible, human beings: update. In: Barrett E (ed) Visions of Rogers' science based nursing. National League for Nursing, New York
Sayre-Adams J, Wright S G 1995 The theory and practice of therapeutic touch. Churchill Livingstone, New York
Taylor B 1994 Being human: ordinariness in nursing. Churchill Livingstone, New York
Woodham A, Peters D 1997 Encyclopaedia of complementary medicine. Dorling Kindersley, London

Wright S G, Sayre-Adams J 2000 Sacred space: right relationship, spirituality and health. Churchill Livingstone, Edinburgh
Young M 1995 Cited in Forder E, Forder J 1995 The light within. Usha Dent
Zohar D 1990 The quantum self. William Morrow, New York

USEFUL ADDRESS

For further information on TT and courses run in the UK:
The Sacred Space Foundation, Ravenscroft, Renwick, Cumbria CA 10 1JL, UK
tel: 01768 898375/fax: 01768 898874
email: Jeannie@sacredspace.org.uk
website: http://www.sacredspace.org.uk

Research

SECTION CONTENTS

11

Non-specific factors in randomized clinical trials: some methodological considerations

Anton J. M. De Craen, Angela J. E. M. Lampe-Schoenmaeckers and Jos Kleijnen

Editor's note

Anton de Craen's study tried to find out whether identical-appearing tablets become more or less effective depending on whether a positive or neutral attitude is expressed by the practitioner giving them. In fact, contrary to what they expected, this appeared not to influence the results. This led them to believe that expectancy must be only one among many significant non-specific factors that influence outcome. The researchers believe that practitioners need to know more about these factors, and that therefore we should develop the kind of research that can identify all the circumstances that determine a maximal treatment effect. We can only agree with the authors that this is an important issue, given what Angela Clow tells us in her chapter about the beneficial physiological changes that result when these circumstances are working well. The chapter raises important questions about how to research the impact of beliefs and the whole range of influences highlighted by our previous authors.

The 1948 trial of streptomycin for the treatment of pulmonary tuberculosis is generally considered to be the first randomized clinical trial (Streptomycin in Tuberculosis Trials Committee 1948). Although other trials have been reported earlier, the trial certainly heralded in a new era in clinical medicine (Vandenbroucke 1987). Until then, most therapies were not judged to be efficacious on the basis of documented observations and comparisons but on pathophysiological rationales provided by authoritative experts (Feinstein 1985). The major advantage of randomized experiments over uncontrolled treatment evaluations is that, on average, at baseline prognostically equivalent groups are generated. After giving active treatment to one group and control treatment to the other, the effect of the intervention can be compared between the two groups. Any difference in result between the two groups can be attributed to the intervention if the following two conditions are satisfied: (1) both groups should have been treated equally after randomization except for the randomized treatment contrast, and (2) outcome assessment should have been performed identically in both groups. These two conditions are not easy to accomplish if a particular intervention is compared with no treatment. A placebo or 'sham' intervention can then be used, which helps to mask the treatment allocation. Hence, use of a placebo intervention can eliminate the subjective effects of the treatment and the effects of intended and unintended behavioural changes. Furthermore, outcome assessment in both groups will not be biased by knowledge of the treatment allocation.

After World War II, randomized clinical trials became the standard method for evaluating treatment effects. Whenever possible, placebo groups were included in experimental designs. In this period, the late 1940s and early 1950s, physicians and researchers observed that the response in the placebo group of a trial was frequently better than one would have thought beforehand. This apparently enhanced response in the placebo group of a trial is usually referred to as the placebo effect. In this chapter we will examine some methodological issues in research of placebo effects.

DEFINITION OF PLACEBO AND PLACEBO EFFECT

The placebo effect has been defined as 'the difference in outcome between a placebo treated group and an untreated control group in an unbiased experiment' (Gøtzsche 1994). Although Gøtzsche stated that it is difficult or impossible to define placebo theoretically, others have pragmatically defined placebo as an empty preparation or intervention imitating an effective preparation or intervention.

Henry Beecher (1955) was one of the first researchers to note the phenomenon of the placebo effect. In his landmark article 'The powerful placebo' he reviewed 15 placebo-controlled trials and concluded that, on average, the magnitude of the placebo effect was 35.2%. In retrospect, the large impact this paper had is difficult to understand as 13 of the 15 papers reviewed did not include no-treatment groups and could therefore not distinguish between changes caused by the natural course of disease and those caused by placebo. Remarkably, in the two studies that did include no-treatment controls no differences were observed between the no-treatment group and the placebo group. Actually, Beecher made the mistake many still make: the observed effect in the placebo group was confused with the placebo effect (Ernst & Resch 1995). The paper has certainly had great impact on the concept of placebo, and might be responsible for the misconception that a fixed fraction (one-third) of patients responds to placebos. It has recently been demonstrated that at least 19 other reasons might be responsible for the changes in the placebo-treated groups of Beecher's review (Kienle 1995). (This was discussed in detail in Ch. 4.)

COLOURED DRUGS AS EXAMPLE OF A PLACEBO EFFECT

Factors such as reputation of the doctor, treatment mode, patient's attitude towards the expected benefit and credibility of the treatment might modify patients' expectancies and hence the therapeutic outcome. Moreover, the colour of a drug formulation might cause different expectations in patients and could therefore produce different therapeutic effects. We have reported a systematic literature review on the colour of drugs where we sought the answers to two questions: (a) are formulations of different colours perceived as equally active and (b) do different-coloured formulations of the same drug produce a different effect in randomized clinical trials (de Craen et al 1996).

Perceived action of coloured drug formulations

We found six publications that studied the perceived action of coloured drugs (Buckalew & Coffield 1982a, b, Buckalew & Ross 1991, Jacobs & Nordan 1979, Sallis & Buckalew 1984, Sebellico 1989). Four studies assessed the expected effect of different colours in terms of stimulant or antidepressant and depressant or tranquillizing (Buckalew & Coffield 1982a, b, Jacobs & Nordan 1979, Sebellico 1989). Red, yellow and orange were related to a stimulant effect, while blue, green and white were associated with a tranquillizing effect (Table 12.1). One study found that the colour of the

Table 12.1   Summary of studies investigating perceived effects of different-coloured drugs

Authors	Blue	Green	Orange	Red	Yellow	White
Buckalew & Coffield 1982a	Depressant	Analgesic	Stimulant	Stimulant		Analgesic
Buckalew & Coffield 1982b	Depressant		Stimulant	Stimulant		
Jacobs & Nordan 1979	Depressant		Stimulant	Stimulant		
Sebellico 1989	Depressant	Depressant	Stimulant	Stimulant	Stimulant	Depressant

Depressant also includes hypnotic and tranquillizing; stimulant includes antidepressant.

drug affected the perceived site of action, white being most common for general drugs, red and scarlet for cardiovascular and blood or lymphatic systems, and tan, beige and burnt orange for skin (Buckalew & Ross 1991). Another investigation studied the perceived strength of coloured capsules. Red and black were perceived as strong and white as weak (Sallis & Buckalew 1984).

Effects of coloured drug formulations

Six trials investigated the influence of the colour of drug formulation on the specific effect (Blackwell, Bloomfield & Buncher 1972, Cattaneo, Luchelli & Filippuci 1970, Huskisson 1974, Luchelli, Cattaneo & Zattoni 1978, Nagao et al 1968, Schapira et al 1970). The methodological quality of these trials, assessed using a previously reported 10-point rating scale (Kleijnen et al 1994), was seven points for two trials (Cattaneo, Luchelli & Filippuci 1970, Schapira et al 1970), six and a half points for one trial (Blackwell, Bloomfield & Buncher 1972), and less than five points for three trials (Huskisson 1974, Luchelli, Cattaneo & Zathoni 1978, Nagao et al 1968). All trials had different designs and different outcome measurements, so a meta-analysis was not possible. Overall, the results indicated differences between colours, but a consistent trend could not be detected. To give an impression of the type of studies that have been carried out, three examples follow.

In a double-blind crossover study, Cattaneo, Luchelli & Filippuci (1970) gave orange and blue placebos to 120 in-patients awaiting minor surgery who thought that they were receiving tranquillizers. In an analysis that excluded patients with no preference, they showed that 26 out of 42 men (62%) preferred orange whereas 33 out of 54 women (61%) preferred blue capsules. Furthermore, they reported that the efficacy data were consistent with the expressed preference.

In a randomized crossover study reported by Luchelli, Cattaneo & Zattoni (1978), 96 patients admitted for elective surgery were randomized to receive either a hypnotic agent or placebo on the first night. On the second night all patients received the other study drug, which was the same colour as that on the night before. Two colours were tested: blue and orange. Patients taking blue capsules reported falling asleep significantly more quickly than those taking the orange capsules (103 minutes versus 135 minutes; $P < 0.05$), and those taking the blue capsules slept for longer (379 minutes versus 346 minutes; $P < 0.01$).

In a crossover trial reported by Huskisson (1974) 24 patients with rheumatoid arthritis received red, blue, green or yellow drugs. Three analgesics were tested against placebo. The red placebo was as effective as any of the active drugs in relieving pain. Blue and green placebos were average pain relievers. Colour did not change the effectiveness of the active drugs.

How can different-coloured drug formulations have different effects?

There might be several explanations why different colours have different effects. Colour itself might have direct psychophysiological effects. Moreover, if the colour of the drug parallels the perceived action then patients might comply better, resulting in a better outcome.

The colour of a drug is not the only perceptual characteristic that could influence patients' response to a drug. Preparation form (capsule or tablet), and size are other factors that may affect a therapeutic response. Buckalew & Coffield (1982) found that capsules are perceived as stronger than tablets. Similarly, in a clinical trial comparing chlordiazepoxide capsules with tablets, Hussain (1972) concluded that in the treatment of anxiety the overall response was better when patients were treated with capsules.

RESEARCH INTO PLACEBO EFFECTS AND INTERNAL VALIDITY

A strong methodological tool for research into placebo effects is the balanced placebo design. In trials with a balanced placebo design patients are randomized to a specific intervention (e.g. administration of medication or placebo) and to a non-specific intervention (e.g. red or white capsules). Using this design it is possible to investigate whether a non-specific factor is capable of modifying the effect of the specific intervention. We have previously reported 10 such trials (Kleijnen et al 1994). Although most of them were considered of limited methodological quality, all indicated different specific effects under the various treatment situations.

We have conducted a placebo-controlled, randomized, double-blind clinical trial with a balanced placebo design within our hospital. The general objective of this trial was to investigate the analgesic effect of tramadol relative to placebo in patients with chronic non-malignant pain, and to investigate whether experimentally induced expectancy could modify this effect. Below we outline a number of important methodological considerations for the design of the trial, type of pharmacologic and nonpharmacologic intervention, and informed consent.

Balanced placebo design

The trial employed a balanced placebo design. Two components were randomly assigned to each patient: the pharmacological intervention (tramadol or placebo) and the non-pharmacological intervention (positive attitude of physician or neutral attitude of physician towards expected benefit of the specific intervention). The first study with this design was reported by Wied in 1953. Wied tried to assess the influence of suggestion on the effects of hormonal therapy compared with a placebo in patients with climacteral complaints. In half of the patients the therapy was given with the suggestion that it concerned a new, expensive, highly effective therapy, whereas the other half was told that it concerned a free-sample preparation of dubious effectiveness. Unfortunately, the effect measurement was also varied in this investigation in a way that in the first group the complaints were assessed in an optimistic tone, whereas in the second group assessment took place in a sceptic tone. If one also takes into account that the placebo was not identical and that the allocation method was not specified, the results (without positive suggestion a clearly larger specific effect) can only be interpreted with caution. According to present standards the study was not well performed and reported.

Pharmacological and non-pharmacological interventions

The pharmacological intervention in the trial was a single oral dose of either tramadol 50 mg or placebo. To match the taste of tramadol, placebo capsules contained 5 mg quinine hydrochloride dihydrate and 10 mg citric acid monohydrate.

The non-pharmacological intervention was a positive attitude expressed by the anaesthesiologist towards the expected effect of tramadol, or a neutral expectancy towards the expected effect. The following statements were used for the positive attitude: 'This is a medication that became recently available in the Netherlands. This drug, according to my experience, is very effective and will decrease the pain quickly after taking it.' In the neutral attitude the following statements were used: 'My own experience with this medication is limited and my impression is that it will not be beneficial in all patients. The pill becomes effective almost immediately, if it is going to have an effect.' These statements were adapted from Gryll & Katahn (1978) who found these statements to give a different response with placebo administration.

Informed consent

Informed consent was obtained for each patient. The information in the informed consent was intended to give each participant a thorough understanding of the nature of the trial and the cooperation required. The following basic elements were included in the informed consent form: (1) a statement that the study involved research and (2) a full and fair explanation of the procedures to be followed.

We considered it essential that patients were not aware of the experimental component of the expectancy manipulation, but we were also aware that we were legally obliged to give all patients a full explanation of the project. We solved this the following way. In the informed consent form it was reported that, apart from the investigation whether tramadol is better than placebo, there was a second objective in the project. In order to be successful, we stated that it was important that participants did not know the nature of this objective. If they were anxious to know what this objective was, they could ask their physician. The physician would then disclose the second objective, after which it was still possible to participate in the trial.

The text of the informed consent was as follows:

Dear madam/sir

We hereby ask your cooperation for a clinical trial investigating the efficacy of a pain killer, tramadol. Below is a description of the trial.

In case you decide to participate in this investigation, your doctor will give you a small capsule. You are requested to take this capsule immediately. Half of the patients will receive tramadol and the other half will receive a placebo (a placebo is a dummy pill). Treatment allocation is random. Moreover, neither the doctor nor you is aware whether you are allocated to the pain killer or the placebo. After you have taken the medication, your normal visit with your doctor will follow. After your visit you are requested to stay within the hospital for about 45 minutes. During this time a research assistant will ask you a number of questions regarding your pain complaints. You will also receive a form on which you can indicate your pain intensity until 24 hours after intake.

Next to the question whether tramadol is better than placebo, there is another question involved in this research. It is important that you do not know beforehand what this question is about. This part of the research is absolutely not harmful. If you want to know what the second research objective is about, you can ask your doctor. In that case we will give you the details of this extra objective after which you can still take part in the investigation. Participation in this research is voluntary. This means that you can make the choice whether or not to participate in this research. Should you decide not to participate, this will by no means affect your treatment in our hospital.

At the beginning of your visit your doctor will ask you whether you are willing to participate in this scientific research. This research is being conducted by the Department of Anaesthesiology in cooperation with the Department of Clinical Epidemiology and Biostatistics of the Academic Medical Centre. The Medical Ethics Committee has approved this research.

Of course we can do this research only with your consent. We hope you understand the research and are willing to help us to carry it out. All information we collect for this research will be treated confidentially and processed anonymously. You can withdraw from this research at any time. If you decide to participate, your doctor will ask you to confirm this by signing an informed consent form.

Primary outcome measures and statistical analysis

Pain intensity was measured using a 10-cm visual analogue scale (VAS), on which the endpoints were marked as no pain (0) and very severe pain (10).

It has been demonstrated that a 10-cm VAS is an appropriate scale to measure self-reported pain intensity in chronic pain patients (Jensen, Turner & Romano 1994). 'Pain intensity difference' was defined as the difference between baseline pain intensity and a subsequent pain intensity measurement. The 'sum pain intensity difference' was calculated as the sum of the pain intensity differences noted at different time points in the postdrug period.

Pain intensity was measured 30 minutes and 60 minutes after randomization. These measurements were carried out by a research fellow who was blinded with regard to the pharmacological intervention, non-pharmacological intervention and baseline pain intensity score. Pain intensity was also assessed by the patient at 2, 4, 6, 8 and 24 hours after randomization. These pain intensity measurements were recorded on a case record form which was mailed to the investigator within 3 days.

The sum of the pain intensity differences at 30 minutes and 60 minutes was the primary outcome variable. All data were analysed using the 'intention to treat' principle. The observed difference between tramadol and placebo in the positive attitude group (dp) was compared with the observed difference between tramadol and placebo in the neutral attitude group (dn). Then dp = dn was tested.

We were not able to demonstrate a different specific effect of tramadol in the positive-attitude group as compared with the neutral-attitude group.

CONCLUSION

Variation in treatment effects between clinical trials is frequently observed. These differences are usually attributed to different patient characteristics, variations in outcome assessment and random error. We think that part of the variation between trials can also be caused by non-specific factors, such as colour of medication or attitude of the treating physician. We were not able to demonstrate any influence of the attitude of the treating physician on the specific effect of tramadol in our trial. However, we think that this does not mean that the phenomenon does not exist; we have probably chosen a wrong model to demonstrate it. In the future, several studies will have to be carried out to reveal which non-specific factors strongly interact with specific treatments. The characteristics of the non-specific factors that define the interaction effects should then be identified. Then for all interventions optimal circumstances in which a maximal treatment effect can be obtained should be assessed, which will lead to a more elaborate research methodology that takes into account the effect modifiers.

We hope that this example will motivate other researchers to start up similar projects. We feel there is a need for several investigations to demonstrate that this is an important topic. Once there is a general agreement that this is the case, a major research effort is necessary to identify the most important non-specific factors, to uncover the mechanisms of action and to assess the methodological implications and the implications for medical practice.

REFERENCES

Beecher H K 1955 The powerful placebo. Journal of the American Medical Association 159:1602–1606
Blackwell B, Bloomfield S S, Buncher C R 1972 Demonstration to medical students of placebo responses and non-drug factors. Lancet i:1279–1282
Buckalew L W, Coffield K E 1982a An investigation of drug expectancy as a function of capsule color and size and preparation form. Journal of Clinical Psychopharmacology 2:245–248
Buckalew L W, Coffield K E 1982b Drug expectations associated with perceptual characteristics: ethnic factors. Perceptual and Motor Skills 55:915–918
Buckalew L W, Ross S 1991 Medication property effects on expectations of action. Drug Development Research 23:101–108
Cattaneo A D, Lucchelli P E, Filippuci G 1970 Sedative effects of placebo treatment. European Journal of Clinical Pharmacology 3:43–45
de Craen A J M, Ross P J, de Vries A L, Kleijnen J 1996 Effect of colour of drugs: systematic review of perceived effect of drugs and of their effectiveness. British Medical Journal 313:1624–1626
Ernst E, Resch K L 1995 Concept of true and perceived placebo effects. British Medical Journal 311:551–553
Feinstein A R 1985 Clinical epidemiology. The architecture of clinical research. W B Saunders, Philadelphia
Gøtzsche P C 1994 Is there logic in the placebo? Lancet 344:925–926
Gryll S L, Katahn M 1978 Situational factors contributing to the placebo effect. Psychopharmacology 47:253–261
Huskisson E 1974 Simple analgesics for arthritis. British Medical Journal iv:196–200
Hussain M Z 1972 Effect of shape of medication in treatment of anxiety states. British Journal of Psychiatry 120:507–509
Jacobs K W, Nordan P M 1979 Classification of placebo drugs: effect of color. Perceptual and Motor Skills 49:367–372
Jensen M P, Turner J A, Romano J M 1994 What is the maximum number of pain levels needed in pain intensity measurement? Pain 58:387–392
Kienle G S 1995 Der sogenannte Placeboeffekt: Illusion, Fakten, Realitat. Schattauer, Stuttgart
Kleijnen J, de Craen A J M, van Everdingen J J E, Krol L J 1994 Placebo effect in double-blind clinical trials: a review of interactions with medication. Lancet 344:1347–1349
Lucchelli P E, Cattaneo A D, Zattoni J 1978 Effect of capsule colour and order of administration of hypnotic treatments. European Journal of Clinical Pharmacology 13:153–155
Nagao Y, Komiya J, Kuroyanagi K, Minaba Y, Susa A 1968 Effect of the color of analgesics on their therapeutic results. Shikwa Gakuho 68:139–142
Sallis R E, Buckalew L W 1984 Relation of capsule color and perceived potency. Perceptual and Motor Skills 58:897–898
Schapira K, McClelland H A, Griffiths M R, Newell D J 1970 Study on the effects of tablet colour in the treatment of anxiety states. British Medical Journal ii:446–449
Sebellico A 1989 11 colore de farmaco: inchiesta preliminare. Bolletino Societa Italiana Biologia Sperimentale 65:685–687
Streptomycin in Tuberculosis Trials Committee 1948 Streptomycin treatment of pulmonary tuberculosis. British Medical Journal ii:769–782
Vandenbroucke J P 1987 A short note on the history of the randomized controlled trial. Journal of Chronic Disease 40:985–987
Wied G L 1953 Ober die bedeutung der Suggestion in der Therapie von klimakterischen Ausfallbeschwerden. Artzl Wochenschrift 8:623–625

12

The placebo effect and a participatory world view

John Heron

Editor's note

I wanted to include a viewpoint that I believe can help us make sense of the paradox of the placebo effect, which has become such a problem for modern medicine and for research. Might it be less of a problem for our practitioner authors precisely because they do not assume a separated mind and body? To a theorist like Hellman or a practitioner like Steve Wright we live in a fundamentally relational world, but how can research design take account of this seamlessness? It means that when researching into self-healing responses we cannot avoid, whether as researchers or 'subjects' of research, being necessarily involved in determining the outcome. And, since we are doing something to the process and outcome of the very thing we are trying to study, we must consider how to judge the quality of our doing and being. I turned to John Heron and asked him to suggest a design that could draw out and take account of factors influencing these mysterious self-healing outcomes. John is an applied philosopher who has helped shape an emerging participatory worldview. Because it is systemic, holistic, relational and experiential, it can lay claim to being a more adequate and creative paradigm for our times. It competes with both modern positivism and with the extreme relativism of the deconstructive post-modern alternative. The worldview is 'participatory' in that it views our world as consisting not of separate things but of relationships; relationships we co-author. And it places human persons and communities as part of a world which we co-create and in which we are embodied. What is more, our co-evolution with the world means that (as Gregory Bateson once put it) mind and nature are necessarily a unity. This has definite implications for any research into the self-healing response because the effect itself is a very mysterious example of how we participate in creating our own world. The participatory worldview and its radical approach to a science of experience is very much Heron's territory and his chapter points to an important way forward for exploring the self-healing response.

INQUIRY PARADIGMS

Any method of inquiry presupposes an inquiry paradigm. This implies and depends on a set of basic beliefs about the nature of reality and how this reality can be known (Guba & Lincoln 1994, Heron & Reason 1997). These are the philosophical presuppositions of a method that are not derived from the method itself and inevitably the continued use of the method will show up the limitations of its underlying paradigm. The implicit beliefs within any such inquiry paradigm can be revealed by three fundamental and interrelated questions:

- the ontological question—'What is the form and nature of reality?
- the epistemological question—'What is the relationship between the knower and reality, and the extent of our knowledge of reality?
- the methodological question—'How can inquirers find out about whatever they believe can be known?'

This chapter will look at the participatory world view in the light of these questions, consider the implications of this world view for our understanding of the body, illness and disease, and explore how a participatory world view would impact on the future of medical practice and research. The concluding focus of this chapter is the outline of a project that would use the participatory research method of cooperative inquiry to elucidate the elements and patterns relevant to the placebo response. But first I want to consider the paradigm presupposed by conventional medical inquiry, and the limitations that have already been revealed by continued use of this approach.

THE CARTESIAN ANOMALY

The inquiry paradigm underlying conventional medicine and mainstream medical research is cartesian and it is fraught with the basic anomaly of

Descartes' dualism. Within this world view, mind and matter are considered to be independent substances, with mind conceived as non-spatial with none of the properties of matter, whereas matter has spatial properties with none of the qualities of mind. The tangible human physical body is included within the self-contained mechanism of the spatially extended material world. This is the world of objects: a real world independent of our minds, operating according to causal laws, which we can find out about by observing how its component parts work together. Such is the objectivist, positivist world view of modern times, which Skolimowski (1994) calls Mechanos. It is the legacy not only of Descartes, but also of Bacon, Galileo and Newton.

The anomaly in Descartes' thinking is that, on the one hand, mind is non-spatial with no bodily properties at all, yet on the other hand he says that the mind is very closely united with the body and as it were intermingled with it (1641). Indeed, he makes the anomaly very specific by saying that the mind interacts with the body through the pineal gland. So, without apparently realizing the difficulty, he gives the non-spatial mind a precise spatial location in the body. Modern medicine perpetuates its own version of this anomaly. This is typified by its use of drugs, chemical substances conceived of as having an independent effect within the assumed autonomous mechanism of the body. The foundation of clinical practice is a view of the body as a self-contained physical system. With its 'therapy hat on', modern medicine wants to deliver purely physical remedies for what it assumes to be purely physical defects. Yet with its 'research hat on', it also has to acknowledge and allow for the dynamic influence of mental belief on this mechanism, which it names the placebo effect. For the guiding rule of effective and reliable medical research—and the very reason for controlling for the placebo effect by experimental design—is that the body is not a self-contained physical system but one that is pervaded by and subject to the influence of mental events.

This is indeed a weird anomaly: the proven effect of mental belief on bodily functioning—the placebo effect—is acknowledged only so that it can be discounted in research and ignored in clinical practice. Thus a remarkable and undisputed healing effect of unknown potential is dealt with in pejorative terms and cast aside as an irrelevant distraction from the pursuit of competent medicine. Harvard Medical School anthropologist Arthur Kleinman asks (de Cuevas 1995): Why is the placebo regarded as pejorative? Is it threatening to medicine? Clearly it is, for it threatens the positivist, objectivist, mechanistic paradigm that underpins both medical research and practice; and hence it subverts the unexamined acceptance of a powerful, unilateral, external control over people's bodies that medicine claims.

I believe the paradigm is cracking up under the strain of that threat. Because a human body is not just an objective reality, part of the autonomous furniture of the universe; it is a subjective–objective reality. That means it is experienced from within and observed from without and therefore when it is dysfunctional there will be both interior experiential illness and exterior observable disease process. But cartesian medicine attends exclusively to the latter while expecting its patient to keep the former out of the doctor's way. But an increasing number of patients, no longer content to skulk passively within their observable bodies and let them be subject purely to external medical control, want to become active agents within their experiential bodies, which are potentially subject to their own control, as the placebo response implies.

THE DOWNFALL OF POSITIVISM

Medical science is one of the human sciences, and the limits of objectivist, quantitative research in the other human sciences have been well reviewed for many years (Argyris 1968, 1970, Bernstein 1983, Gergen 1973, Guba & Lincoln 1994, Harrè & Secord 1972, Heather 1976, Israel & Tajfel 1972, Joynson 1974, Lincoln & Guba 1985, Reason & Rowan 1981, Shotter 1975, Smith, Harrè & Van Langenhove 1995). I will give here a brief summary of some of the main criticisms.

The overarching criticism is that there is no external world entirely independent of the researcher's mind against which to verify or falsify hypotheses:

• The findings of the observer are shaped by the observer in interaction with the phenomena observed. This is evident both in the physical and the social sciences.

• Statements of so-called 'objective fact' are theory laden, for they can be formulated only within a pre-existing set of theoretical assumptions.

• These same statements of fact are also value laden, for the underlying theoretical assumptions that shape them represent values preferred to other values implicit in other rejected assumptions.

More specific criticisms relate to quantitative approaches that use inferential statistics, the control of selected variables through randomized designs and imported categories of understanding. Their relevance to medical research is no less telling than it is in the other human sciences (Heron 1986, 1996).

Selecting and controlling variables means the exclusion of others that are influential, and can involve discounting some of those that are selected and controlled. Consequently the resulting findings have little relevance to understanding the real world where all the pertinent variables may be at work. This problem is endemic in medical research, which is designed to discount the influential variable of the placebo effect. The result is that modern medicine has no systematic grasp whatsoever of how the effect of mental attitude on bodily processes is at work in the real world of clinical practice.

Inferential statistics bury individual differences under comparisons of means, and throw no light on the idiosyncratic nature of individual responses. In medical research, the results of clinical trials imply a homogeneity of their research populations. The statistical method used hides what happens to individuals in the trial. With respect to two treatment groups, statistical analysis may show that one treatment is better than another, although there may for instance be some people in both groups who are worse after treatment. In general, medical research works to obscure rather than illuminate interactive effects between treatments and personal characteristics (Weinstein 1974). It can throw no light on the fact that individuals respond differently to the same treatment. Therefore it cannot help with the everyday clinical question: 'What is the treatment of choice for this individual patient?' There is thus a mismatch between research method and clinical reality. The former assumes that patients are the same and obscures their differences, whereas the latter repeatedly reveals the differences amongst patients that defeat this assumption. The inevitable result is a therapeutic culture that has a significant iatrogenic effect. Treatment based on conventional inferential statistics is bound sooner or later to harm some patients in ways that medical research can neither predict nor understand.

People cannot be adequately understood either in terms of externally measured variables or in terms of researcher-imported categories. A full understanding of people necessarily includes the meanings and purposes they invest in their way of being and their actions, as these are interpreted through dialogue with them. Yet medical research totally ignores the meanings and purposes that people invest in their experiential illnesses and attends exclusively to their observable diseases. By ignoring what I will call the 'intentionality' of illness—by which I mean the way people choose to feel it, construe it and enact it—medical culture systematically and continuously disempowers people by regarding their subjectivity as irrelevant to their healing.

The methodology presupposes strict causal determinism. A model of relative indeterminism and autonomous agency is better suited to the explanation of human behaviour. Medical culture treats people as patients contained within bodies subject to strict causal determinism, and as recipients of external therapeutic control. However, the placebo effect suggests, on the contrary, that people are autonomous agents who have within them the power to influence what goes on in their bodies. Such processes are therefore relatively indeterministic, or (which is the same thing) are only relatively determined by causal laws at the purely physical level.

A PARTICIPATORY WORLD VIEW

Not only in medical research, but also in the other academic human sciences, in consciousness research, subatomic physics, systems research, ecology and so on, the distinction between the subjective and the objective is becoming ever more blurred. In many fields the inquiry paradigm of objectivist Mechanos is failing to do justice to the full range of human experience. An emerging alternative inquiry paradigm is that of participative reality. While this accepts that there is a given cosmos, it also holds that the mind participates in it creatively, and that it can only know this cosmos in terms of constructs. These constructs can be experiential, imaginal, conceptual or practical. We can know that we are in touch with what is other only through an active participation of mind, articulated through the use of all our mental sensibilities. Reality is subjective–objective: our own constructs clothe a felt participation in what is present. To touch, see or hear something or someone does not tell us either about our self all on its own, nor about a thing or being out there all on its own; it tells us about a thing or being in a state of interrelation and copresence with us. Worlds and people are what we meet, but the meeting is shaped by our own terms of reference (Bateson 1979, Heron 1992, 1996, Merleau-Ponty 1962, Reason 1994a, Reason & Rowan 1981, Spretnak 1991, Skolimowski 1994, Varela, Thompson & Rosch 1993). The participatory paradigm asserts that we cannot have any final or absolute experience of what there is because, in the relation of knowing by face-to-face acquaintance, the experiential knower shapes perceptually what is out there.

The point about experiential knowing is that the very process of perceiving is also a meeting, a transaction. To experience anything is to participate in it, and to participate is both to mould and to encounter. When I hold your hand, I both subjectively shape you and objectively meet you. To encounter being or a being is both to image it in my way and to know that it is out there. Hence experiential reality is always subjective–objective. It is subjective because it is known only through the form the mind, perceptually and conceptually, gives it, and it is objective because the mind penetrates a cosmos that it shapes.

Merleau-Ponty (1964, p. 317) shows how perception itself is participatory so that:

in so far as my hand knows hardness and softness, and my gaze knows the moon's light, it is as a certain way of linking up the phenomena and communicating with it. Hardness and softness, roughness and smoothness, moonlight and sunlight, present themselves in our recollection not pre-eminently as sensory contents but as certain kinds of symbioses, certain ways the outside has of invading us and certain ways we have of meeting the invasion.

Or, as Skolimowski puts it: 'Things become what our consciousness makes of them through the active participation of our mind' (1994, pp. 27–28).

Bateson (in Brockman 1977, p. 245) makes the point that between the extremes of solipsism, in which 'I make it all up', and a purely external reality, in which I cease to exist, there is: 'a region where you are partly blown by the winds of reality and partly an artist creating a composite out of inner and outer events'.

From all this it follows that what can be known about the given cosmos is that it is always known as a subjectively articulated world, whose objectivity is relative to how it is shaped by the knower. But this is not all: its objectivity is also relative to how it is intersubjectively shaped. For there is the important if obvious point that knowers can only be knowers when known by other knowers: knowing presupposes mutual participative awareness. It presupposes participation, through meeting and dialogue, in a culture of shared art and shared language, shared values, norms and beliefs. And, deeper still, agreement about the rules of language, about how to use it, presupposes a tacit mutual experiential knowing and understanding between people that is the primary ground of all explicit forms of knowing (Heron 1996). So any subjective–objective reality articulated by any one person is done within an intersubjective field, a context of shared meanings—at one level linguistic–cultural and, at a deeper level, experiential.

FOUR WAYS OF KNOWING

At this point we should recall the epistemological question: 'What is the relationship between the knower and reality, and the extent of our knowledge of reality?' A participative world view, with its notion that reality is subjective–objective, involves an extended epistemology (Heron 1992, 1996). Reflecting on what and how we know, it becomes clear that the knower participates in the known, and articulates and shapes a world, in at least four interdependent ways. These ways are experiential, presentational, propositional and practical: four ways of knowing that constitute the spectrum of our subjectivity. Within it we have enormous latitude to acknowledge its components and utilize them in association, or to dissociate from them and disintegrate them from each other. Therefore this epistemology presents us as knowers with an interesting developmental challenge: that of critical subjectivity. This involves an awareness of the four ways of knowing, and of how they are currently interacting. Furthermore it implies ways of changing the relations between these ways so that they articulate a subjective–objective reality unclouded by a restrictive and ill-disciplined subjectivity.

Experiential knowing

Experiential knowing means direct encounter, face-to-face meeting, feeling and imaging the presence of some energy, entity, person, place, process or thing. It is knowing through participative, empathic resonance with a being, so that as knower I feel both attuned with it yet distinct from it. It is also the creative shaping of a world through the transaction of imaging it, perceptually and in other ways. Experiential knowing thus articulates reality through felt resonance with the inner being of what is there, and through perceptually enacting (Varela, Thompson & Rosch 1993) its forms of appearing.

Presentational knowing

Presentational knowing emerges from and is grounded on experiential knowing, and clothes it in the metaphors of aesthetic creation. It expresses the primary meaning embedded in our experiential, enacted knowing and symbolizes it in graphic, plastic, musical, vocal, choreographic and verbal art-forms.

Propositional knowing

Propositional knowing is knowing in conceptual terms that something is the case and is ultimately grounded in our experiential articulation of a world. It is knowledge by description of some energy, entity, person, place, process or thing expressed in statements and theories that come with the mastery of concepts and classes that language bestows. Its propositions are carried by presentational forms in the sounds or visual shapes of the spoken or written word.

Practical knowing

Practical knowing is knowing how to do something, demonstrated in a skill or competence, and is in an important sense primary (Heron 1996). It presupposes a conceptual grasp of principles and standards of practice, and involves presentational elegance, experientially grounded in the situation within which the action occurs. It fulfils these three prior forms of knowing, bringing them to fruition in purposive deeds: it consummates them in an autonomous celebration of excellent accomplishment. It not only consummates them, but is also grounded in them. (The bipolar relationship is presented diagrammatically in Fig. 13.1.)

CRITICAL SUBJECTIVITY

Critical subjectivity means that we attend both to the grounding relations between the forms of knowing and also to their consummating relations. Through primary subjective experiential knowing we articulate our being in a world. As such it is the ground of the other forms of knowing but, naively exercised, it is likely to be distorted by defensive and collusive

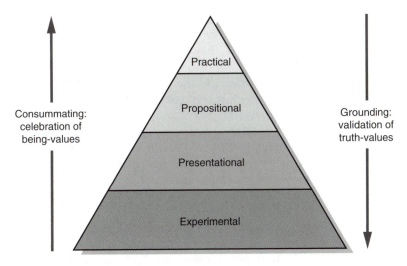

Consummating:
celebration of
being-values

Practical

Propositional

Presentational

Experimental

Grounding:
validation of
truth-values

Figure 13.1   Bipolar congruence of four forms of knowing.

processes. By attending to subjective experience with a critical consciousness, we may bring it into aware relation with the other three ways of knowing. These clarify and refine and elevate it at the same time as more adequately grounding it. Only when there is congruence between the four aspects of knowing can there be a claim to validity. In addition, since our knowing is from a perspective then when we are aware of that perspective, of its authentic value and of its restricting bias we articulate this awareness in our communications. Critical subjectivity involves this self-reflexive attention to the ground on which one is standing. It also extends to critical intersubjectivity. Since our personal knowing is always set within a context of linguistic–cultural and experiential shared meaning, having a critical consciousness about our knowing necessarily includes dialogue, feedback and exchange with others. This leads to the methodology of cooperative inquiry.

METHODOLOGY OF COOPERATIVE INQUIRY

Let us remind ourselves of the methodological question: 'How can inquirers find out about whatever they believe can be known?' The inquiry method within a participative world view needs to draw on the four ways of knowing in a way that ensures critical subjectivity will be enhanced by critical intersubjectivity. It aims to be a form of research acknowledging that all involved are both researchers and subjects. Together they engage in democratic dialogue as coresearchers to design, manage and draw conclusions from the research. And as cosubjects they engage in the action and experience that is the focus of the research (Heron 1971, 1981a, b, 1985,

1988, 1992, 1996, 1998, 2000, Heron & Reason 1986, 1997, 2000, Reason 1988a, 1994a, b, Reason & Heron 1995). In such cooperative inquiry people collaborate to agree the questions they want to explore and to define their method for that exploration (propositional knowing). Together or separately they apply this methodology to the world of their practice (practical knowing), which leads to new forms of encounter with their world (experiential knowing); and they find ways to represent this experience in significant patterns (presentational knowing), which in turn feeds into a revised propositional understanding of the originating questions. Together coinquirers cycle several times through the four forms of knowing in order to move, over successive cycles, from experience of a topic to shared reflection on it, which revises the way they will next explore it experientially, and so on.

Research cycling is a primary way of enhancing critical subjectivity and the validity of inquirers' claims to have articulated a subjective–objective reality. A range of further procedures aimed at developing this effect include: managing divergence and convergence within and between cycles; balancing reflection and action; securing authentic collaboration; challenging uncritical subjectivity and intersubjectivity; managing unaware projections and displaced anxiety; and attending to the dynamic interplay of chaos and order. These are mentioned in a little more detail later on. For a full discussion, together with a set of radical skills of being and doing required during the action phases of the inquiry, and for a comprehensive account of cooperative inquiry see Heron (1996).

THE BODY AS A SUBJECTIVE–OBJECTIVE REALITY

A human body is par excellence not something 'out there' in the world, independent of human subjectivity. It is a participatory reality, a subjective–objective reality, and the most basic sense in which this is so is in my knowing of my own body. In terms of the fourfold epistemology outlined earlier, the grounding knowing of my body is in terms of experiential knowing, whose basis is proprioception: feeling from within the movement, posture and qualitative state of my body. This inner felt sense is the spatiotemporal foundational knowing of my body as extended in space, moving—and pulsing rhythmically—in time. It is elaborated by how I image my body in all other sensory modalities—that is, by touching and seeing it and hearing it. For the participatory world view, my body is a reality that partially consists of my internal experience of it. I will call this inner felt sense of embodiment the 'experiential body'. And the experiential body to some degree shapes the given body; this is the subjective–objective reality of the human body.

A polar, complementary way of knowing the given body is by external observation, elaborated by a whole range of physical instruments and interventions, and symbolized by verbal and numerical statements. This 'observable body—as it is known in natural science—is certainly not the given body in some external, absolute, objective sense. It is the given body as shaped by, and relative to, our observing and cognitive capacities in interaction with it. Therefore the observable body is also a subjective–objective reality. But the observable body may provide us with some grasp of how far the experiential body shapes the given body. We can use this as an external marker of the interaction, but cautiously, because the sensibilities and modes of cognition we deploy in framing the observable body in part constitute it. Always remembering this, we can talk for convenience of how the experiential body does or does not shape the observable body.

Formative intentionality of the experiential body

The inner felt sense of my body is not merely passive receptivity. It is active–passive, intentional–responsive, depending on how I (with greater or lesser awareness) intend it. I shape my body by how I move, gesture, posture, breathe and make sound, by how I qualitatively experience it, how I value and invest meaning in it, and by how I image it in other sensory modalities. All these things all the time are intentional, chosen, however relatively unaware that choice may be. For example I may have made some adaptive survival choices early in my life, which became so habitual that I have lost any sense of their being choices and so I kid myself they are just my given body. But that they are choices becomes clear if I realize that I can unchoose them and become awarely purposive about changing the way I 'do', be in and shape my body. Furthermore, every subtle microchoice about how I 'do' my embodiment is a preference for one way of doing it over another. Each such preference is an embodiment of one emotional value favoured over another that is discarded. In the participatory world view, all these things—how I move, gesture, posture, breathe, make sound, how I qualitatively experience my body, emotionally value and invest meaning in it, image it in other sensory modalities—shape what I come to know analytically and propositionally about my body. What none of us yet know in any great detail is how much we do and might shape the externally observable body. Hence the significance of the new area of psychoneuroimmunology (Watkins 1997).

Formative intentionality of illness and of recreating wellness

It follows from all the above that any observable disease process is, from the standpoint of the participatory paradigm, shaped—at least in part—by its correlative subjective experiential illness: by how people are spatio-temporally doing and being in their body, investing emotional value and meaning in it, imaging in all sensory modalities their experiential body. Yet the still prevalent dualistic paradigm creates a cultural climate in which people continually discount the ways in which the unacknowledged intentionality of their illness is to some degree shaping their externally observable disease.

One reason that patients occlude this inner intentionality is because, by relying on the external authority of the doctor (and the disempowering propositional knowledge of a medical culture), they tend to relinquish any sense of themself as an agent. The question whether their subjective experience of illness is affecting the disease process simply does not arise and so the unknown capacity to change this process remains unexercised and unexplored.

But if my subjective experience of illness is implicitly intentional and if it in part shapes observable disease, then raising consciousness about this and being explicitly intentional with full awareness about how I am spatiotemporally doing, emotionally valuing and meaning my embodiment, may have the potential to reshape observable disease. The hypothesis would be that it would be possible to set out to change the experiential illness into experiential wellness and thereby to modify observable disease processes. This would be intentional self-healing. Its potential capacity is at present unknown, so the implications of the participatory paradigm need to be used with consideration and caution. We are not entitled to make people with diseases feel inadequate and guilty by telling them dogmatically that their diseases are even partly the effects of their unowned states of mind. The most we are entitled to do is put forward the hypothesis that it may to some degree be such a product, and to invite those for whom this idea seems plausible and relevant to engage with their own condition and explore it in active practice.

Symbolizing the experiential body

Everything that anyone comes to know about the observable body in terms of propositional knowledge—anatomy, biochemistry, physiology, aetiology and pathology—rests on and presupposes the subjective experience of indwelling a body. This subjective knowing necessarily forever falls outside the terms and methods of the external observation. In short, my experiential body is the ground of but is irreducible to my knowledge of the observable body. This felt experience of indwelling a body cannot be described in statements based on external, analytic observation. For instance statements in terms of kinaesthetic relays from neural sites in the joints, muscles and so on neither describe it nor explain it. They only provide details of its biomechanical concomitants.

In terms of fourfold knowing, the experiential body is first and foremost symbolized most accessibly through my movement, posture, gesture and mode of breathing. These presentational forms, with their own inherent emotional meaning, directly convey how I am embodying myself. So in order to raise my awareness about the sort of tacit intentionality at work in my experiential body I have to begin to notice how I am choosing to embody myself: my movement, voice, posture, gesture and breathing. These living symbols tell me about the emotional values and meaning I invest in my being in a body. Out of this awareness of the creative intentionality of the experiential body I might develop a conscious presentational artistry, a form of self-healing expressed in terms of personal embodiment and presence. People may thus choose awarely to symbolize a transformed emotional meaning and value they give to the embodied life of their experiential body. In this scheme of things the foundation of intentional wellness and self-healing has to do with making a radical connectedness between life, motion, spatiotemporal form and rhythm, intentionality and emotional attitude.

The formative power of others' experiential knowing

We inter-act. You participate in the subjective–objective reality of my body by experientially knowing it; by perceptually imaging it and intuiting the meaning of my movements, sounds, postures and gestures, and through empathic resonance with my experience of indwelling it. Because this is a participative knowing of my body, and therefore a subjective–objective transaction, it is to some unknown degree formative. That is to say, as you perceive me and (more or less knowingly but nevertheless inevitably) empathically resonate with my experience, this influences and shapes my subjective–objective bodily reality. This effect may (or may not) be minimal compared with the greater influences of the world around, but for the participatory paradigm it is there. To take a significant example, this means that experiential encounters between medical practitioners and patients will always have some effect both on patients' experience of illness and on their observable disease. The potential exists for practitioners to resonate and attune not only to how people are actually being in their body, but also with their as yet unexplored potential for being in it in creative, transforming ways. The primary impact of the practitioner–patient relationship, according to this view, depends on how the practitioner perceptually images, resonates and is present with the patient, rather than on what is said. But what is said by the practitioner will also have a powerful secondary impact if it is rooted in and emerges from the primary impact of such presence.

SUPPORTIVE DATA

There are a lot of data to support the participatory view of the body as a subjective–objective reality whose intentional subjectivity is in part constitutive of it and has power to some unknown degree to influence its processes. The most immediate example is of course the placebo effect: the fact that the expectation of an effect from an ingested substance or therapeutic transaction can actually produce a bodily effect. But apart from this there is the impact of human intention on bodily processes as mediated externally by biofeedback devices and mediated internally by autogenic training, relaxation, visualization and mediation, or through control of movement and breathing. The powerful influence of posthypnotic suggestion on the reversal of functional and structural bodily disorder is another relevant example. There are also documented cases of attitudinal healing in which an intentional transformation of an internal attitude of mind apparently leads to a reduction or elimination of observable disease process.

There is, in addition, growing support for the participatory view that the experiential encounter between practitioner and patient has an influence on outcomes. For example, medical education and primary care practice now underline the importance and value of the doctor–patient relationship; and studies show significantly different outcomes depending on how it is handled (Cousins 1990). Associated with this is the literature on the value of communication skills as determinants of outcome and related psychotherapeutic research suggesting that it is a therapist's qualities of personal presence (rather than any particular therapeutic techniques) that determine outcomes of the therapeutic interaction.

Perhaps more difficult to explain, but supportive of some kind of participatory resonance between people, is the psychoanalytic literature describing significant empathic communication of unarticulated feelings (see Ch. 8). This may overlap with the practice described by some complementary therapists of using tactile skills such as craniosacral therapy or Therapeutic Touch to produce empathic engagement with patients, which is apparently associated with effective outcomes (see Ch. 11). Other therapists seek a charismatic engagement with patients, claiming this empowers radical lifestyle changes in them.

THE RELEVANCE AND LIMITS OF CONVENTIONAL MEDICAL RESEARCH

All these data—some experimental, most qualitative and descriptive—are sufficiently well documented and creditable to call for further research into the participatory paradigm. The question is: what sort of research? Conventional medical research methods can be, and have been, used with good effect to compare a group of people who have some disease and who practise intentional self-help with matched controls who are having no treatment, or some conventional treatment, or both (Cousins 1990, Spiegel 1993). The use of a controlled trial with random allocation in this area of research entails unavoidable problems, however. First, randomization entails a moral obligation to seek the informed consent of people to participate in the trial, which means asking people to agree to the possibility of being randomly allocated to a control group in which they are not to practise intentional self-healing. Apart from the dubious morality of this request, it is self-defeating, because it is in itself a powerfully paradoxical suggestion. Secondly, when it comes to intentionality, medical research using randomized designs is faced with a dilemma. For although it is clearly necessary for it to attempt some sort of exploration into patient intentionality, by doing so the research implicitly subverts its own epistemology and methodologies. Yet by maintaining its customary perspectives on practice and research it is bound to ignore or disempower the patient intentionality it seeks to understand.

At the very least an appropriate design would have to be non-randomized, perhaps with matched controls selected from the records of centres of excellence. Such a non-randomized approach could yield useful external data whereby observable disease processes in the intentional self-healing group were compared with a no-treatment or conventional-treatment group. However, the use of conventional research design and statistical analysis will always be unable to reveal the features of intentional self-healing in which we are most interested—in particular:

- the internal strategies, the subjective processes of intentional self-healing as such—that is, the practical knowledge involved in knowing how to do it
- individual differences amongst patients with respect to effective strategies
- the therapeutic effect understood as a dynamic pattern of the main influential variables: patient intentionality, psychosocial context, observable disease process, copatient interaction, relationships with healthcare professionals and external remedies and procedures used (Heron 1996).

THE RELEVANCE OF COOPERATIVE INQUIRY

If these issues are to be addressed then we must, in order to achieve the aims of the research, stop thinking of ill people as passive patients. Instead, they have to be invited to join with relevant healthcare professionals and cooperative inquiry initiators and become active as intentional agents in a process of inquiry. The patients involved must be coinquirers as well as cosubjects, since their agency and mental state will be key variables. These variables can be used properly (and their use can be properly understood) only if at the outset patients participate in deciding how and why they are to be used. In other words, self-healing as an intentional process can be researched only by those who are engaging with their own subjectivity and at the same time striving towards a critical subjectivity, as defined earlier.

It should be obvious that factors such as internal agency and the role of self-help, as forms of practical knowing-how, can be investigated only by the agents concerned. These agents must also understand these factors in the context of a total pattern of other influential variables, and grasp what whole pattern makes for a significant effect on both experiential illness and observable disease. The coinquirers come to this understanding through cycles of action and reflection, varying the pattern in the action phases of the inquiry, and learning, in the reflection phases, to discriminate what makes for a healing pattern. Rather than allowing such variables to be split between an experimental and a control group, all of them have to be studied together as a total pattern in the inquiry group. The validity of the pattern is inherent in its organization, which can only be studied from within it (Reason 1986). Such immersion in real-life patterns is potentially confusing for inquirers, and makes it all the more essential that they should collaborate with one another to refine their critical subjectivity—the cornerstone of validity in this research method. Moreover, the experience in previous cooperative inquiries is that members get increasingly involved in understanding the participatory paradigm as a shared world space, an intersubjective way of experiencing and construing reality. The more this world view is made explicit, the more it alerts people to cooperate in empowering their critical subjectivity.

A COOPERATIVE INQUIRY PROJECT EXPLORING SELF-HEALING RESPONSE

Cooperative inquiry has so far been used in the health arena in two ways: among healthcare professionals, of the same or different kinds, looking together at their work; and among peer groups of people with a particular physical or medical condition taking charge of how their condition is defined and treated. To my knowledge there has been no small- or large-scale use of full-blown cooperative inquiry with a group of patients who have been invited to revision themselves as potential self-healing agents and who are coinquirers with their relevant healthcare professionals. For an early proposal about a related project, see Reason & Heron (1986).

This participative medical research project aims to allow the unknown potential of self-healing agency to be explored. The method, while it gives full rein to subjectivity, is none the less rigorous. The project has three intentions: first, that inquirers articulate their reality; secondly, that by doing so through a collaborative process inquirers come to know illness in a participative sense; thirdly, that by knowing it in the fourfold way described they transform the experience of illness, or influence observable disease, or both.

Obstacles to participative medical research

These include the following.

- The inquiry methodology is not well known, nor is its underlying paradigm widely understood.
- The objectivist paradigm strongly resists the idea that there can be any alternative method.
- The participative approach potentially subverts the normal power relations of medicine and positivist research. Forms of participatory research that include patients as self-directed coresearchers threaten the political hegemony of conventional medicine and its tendency to control patients' lives.
- The dominance of the cartesian model of physical medicine as a purely technical project creates a demoralizing and disempowering climate, which undermines people's belief in their potential for self-healing. Patient subjectivity is seen, by both patient and doctor, as an embarrassing irrelevance.
- Medical dualism not only splits mind from body, but implies that some diseases are autonomous incurable faults, independent of our minds and waiting to overcome our bodies. It could be that this threatening notion causes some people, through fear, to induce these very faults mentally. For in the participatory world view we both subjectively and intersubjectively articulate and shape our realities. From this viewpoint it is not simply that the practical application of modern medicine and its research methods inescapably produce iatrogenic effects; rather that its underlying perspectives will to a degree actually paralyse self-healing, perhaps inducing experiential illness and even leading to observable disease.
- A fundamental obstacle is the well-known human resistance to self-development. Those who find it inconvenient or unbearable to notice (much less to own) the negative attitudes that shape their way of being embodied would have to dismantle such denial before beginning intentional transformation.

Membership and roles

For these reasons, patients wanting to join a cooperative inquiry about intentional self-healing need to self-select themselves carefully. Certain qualities would be essential: they must not be too debilitated, be willing to take up the participatory paradigm and to rebuff the dualistic medical model, and be open to inquiry, not deluded by unwarranted assumptions, not too resistant and willing to develop their own practical knowing about how to be embodied.

A cooperative inquiry project about intentional self-healing would involve self-selected patients, relevant healthcare professionals and cooperative inquiry initiators. Everyone in the project would be involved in the thinking and planning that designs the inquiry, managing its ongoing process and drawing conclusions from it. Everyone would also be involved in the action and experience being researched—that is, in the chosen intentional practices, either to transform experiential illness in patient members or to enhance experiential wellness in non-patient members. For the non-patient members cannot properly understand and grasp the nature of, and make decisions about, intentional practices and their dynamic relation to other factors unless they engage in them themselves.

The stages of the project

First reflection meeting

This first reflection might extend over several meetings, which the cooperative inquiry initiators would facilitate and guide so as to support the group in evolving some fundamental concepts, presented in basic English. This would mean the group agreeing a provisional working model of intentional agency, of the other influential variables, and of an effective life-enhancing pattern of interaction among them. The result of this stage of inquiry might for example include tentative models of:

- how human intention and subjectivity may mould bodily process and form
- how to understand the tacit intentionality of experiential illness and its relation to observable disease
- ways to transform experiential illness intentionally into experiential wellness
- ways to enhance experiential wellness
- the influential variables involved, and an effective pattern of their interaction—the variables considered might include: intentional agency (self-help techniques), relevant psychosocial factors, observable bodily process, coagent interaction (between patients, between non-patients, and between patients and non-patients) and external remedies and procedures used.

Criteria for defining and recording the state of the subjective, experiential body of all those involved in the project would also have to be agreed: including the experiential illness of the patients, and the relative experiential wellness of the non-patient members. An account of their external, observable bodies would also have to be made: for instance with regard to the observable disease of the patient members as well as the observable bodily integrity of the non-patient members.

Once all this recording is done the group would agree on the range of self-directed techniques for recovery from illness and for enhancing well-ness, and practise together the skills involved. Ways of monitoring and recording the ongoing use of these techniques and their apparent effects, both subjective and observable, must be agreed too. Inquirers then choose the particular techniques they feel motivated to use in the first phase of the application cycles.

The group members would need also to agree on their time framework: how long each phase of application will be, how long each intervening meeting for review, reflection and further planning will be, and how many cycles of application and reflection there will be overall. During this entire first cycle, all decisions and activities agreed have to be documented. Only once all this has been done can the group embark on the agreed series of inquiry cycles.

Cycles of inquiry

In the first application phase, members would apply their chosen self-directed techniques for intentional self-healing and enhanced well-being in the context of the agreed pattern of other influential factors. They need also to keep records, in ways already agreed, of the use and apparent effects of their activities, and of their contextual pattern.

At the next reflection meeting, all this data would be shared and made sense of within the whole group. In the light of this, group members revise the various decisions made at the first reflection meeting, and plan the next application phase so as to take them into account. And so the coinquirers proceed through the remaining inquiry cycles, moving from application phases to reflection and forward-planning meetings. Progressively, cycle by cycle, group members would modify and extend the use of self-directed techniques, accumulating data about their effects, refining and amending the model of how all the relevant influential factors may fruitfully interact.

Validity in the inquiry

During these cycles, the cooperative inquiry initiators will be prompting the group to take time out to review validity issues (for a full discussion see Heron 1996). They include the following.

 • **Managing divergence and convergence within and between cycles**. This attends to whether people are doing different things (divergence) or the same thing (convergence) within a given application phase; also in a given application phase compared with the previous one. Too much divergence gives only an impressionistic account of the topic as a whole. Too much convergence gives an in-depth account of only one part of the topic, unrelated to other parts.

- **Balancing reflection and action**. This means checking that there is neither too much time spent on application in relation to time spent on reflection, nor vice versa.
- **Securing authentic collaboration**. This is done by attending regularly to the right of each participant to have a genuine say in all aspects of research decision making, and to engage fully in the application phases of the inquiry.
- **Challenging uncritical subjectivity and intersubjectivity**. One basic method is the adoption of some form of devil's advocate procedure in which time is taken by any group member to confront possible collusion, delusion and illusion.
- **Managing unaware projections and displaced anxiety**. This means attending to and clearing emotional and interpersonal distress activated by the inquiry process.
- **Attending to the dynamic interplay of chaos and order**. This involves tolerating phases of uncertainty, disorder and confusion, allowing authentic order to emerge in its own good time out of chaos, without rushing anxiously into premature closure.

Completing the inquiry

The concluding reflection meeting, or series of meetings, will draw together the threads of the inquiry. The objective is for coinquirers—patients and non-patients—to exercise, on the basis of the accumulated experiential data, a final discriminating judgement about any patterns of influential factors that have been effective, and in particular the weight given to the use of intentional self-help techniques compared with other factors. In order to achieve this, all members would record their end-states of experiential illness and experiential wellness, and of observable disease and observable bodily integrity. They would compare these with the opening—and any intermediate—records. Both common and idiosyncratic findings are honoured, for both patient and non-patient members. Similarities and differences—of self-help techniques used, their effects, their relation to other influential factors—between patient and non-patient members of the inquiry will help clarify for both groups an understanding of all these things.

It is important to grasp here that the relevant influential variables cannot be understood by selecting and controlling them, nor by splitting them up between different groups. This procedure would fail to detect a valid effect, which is provided by the interacting pattern of all the variables together. Nor could this pattern be interpreted by someone outside the group seeking to control their total interaction, without selection and splitting, who is not involved in their use. Since the patterns sought include intentional subjectivity, they can only be understood by those who are enacting them—that is, by coresearchers who are also cosubjects. The inability to comprehend this idea is one of the main stumbling blocks for positivist researchers.

Finally the group will refine their practical knowledge of effective intentional self-healing techniques, and prepare some descriptive guidelines for their use. They will refine their original working model of how human intention and subjectivity mould bodily process and form, of the tacit intentionality of experiential illness and its relation to observable disease, of intentional ways of transforming experiential illness into experiential wellness and of enhancing experiential wellness.

Throughout the inquiry process the group's use of critical subjectivity and critical intersubjectivity will have improved. In the light of this learning the group will review the validity of their findings and their use of validity procedures and also plan how to prepare some cooperative report on the whole project. Ultimately all coinquirers would have to read, edit and offer amendments to an initial draft, and eventually agree the final version. However, it is fair to point out that, although a written report is valuable and useful, the primary outcome of the inquiry would be the range of practical knowledge gained by the coinquireres—that is, the skills involved in using intentional self-healing and self-development; and the skills involved in harnessing them within a total pattern of effective life-enhancing endeavour. Furthermore, from the viewpoint of the participatory paradigm, and of subjective–objective reality, any written records have only contextual validity—that is, their validity is relative to the inquiry group that generates them and to its articulation of reality. The findings are not, strictly speaking, generalizable in the traditional positivist sense of external validity. For no matter how substantial and significant they may be they can in effect be no more than guidelines whereby other similar groups with similar interests could devise an action-oriented inquiry to articulate their own reality.

CONCLUSION: APPLYING COOPERATIVE INQUIRY

Cooperative inquiry has been applied in diverse fields to study: altered states of consciousness, black managers and subordinates, child protection supervision, cocounselling, cooperation between conventional and complementary practitioners (Reason 1991), and between dental practitioners, in district council organizational culture, amongst health visitors, obese and postobese women, other people with a particular physical or medical condition taking charge of how their condition is defined and treated, whole person medicine in general practice (Heron & Reason 1985, Reason 1988b), women's staff in a university, young women managers, youth workers and more. For further references see Reason (1988a, 1994a) and Heron (1996). Cooperative inquiry is related to other forms of participative inquiry such as action science (Argyris & Schön 1974, Argyris, Putnam & Smith 1985, Schön 1983), action inquiry (Torbert 1991), participatory action research (Fals-Borda & Rahman 1991), some forms of feminist inquiry (Mies 1993, Olesen 1994), emancipatory action research (Carr & Kemmis 1986), appreciative inquiry (Cooperrider & Srivastva 1987), fourth-generation evaluation (Guba & Lincoln 1989), intervention research (Fryer & Feather 1994) and others. For how these differ from cooperative inquiry see Heron (1996).

REFERENCES

Abram D 1996 The spell of the sensuous. Pantheon, New York
Argyris C 1968 Some unintended consequences of rigorous research. Psychological Bulletin 70:185–197
Argyris C 1970 Intervention theory and method: a behavioural science view. Addison Wesley, Reading, MA
Argyris C, Schön D 1974 Theory in practice: increasing professional effectiveness. Jossey-Bass, San Francisco
Argyris C, Putnam R, Smith M C 1985 Action science: concepts, methods and skills for research and intervention. Jossey-Bass, San Francisco
Bateson G 1979 Mind and nature: a necessary unity. Dutton, New York
Bernstein R J 1983 Beyond objectivism and relativism. Basil Blackwell, Oxford
Bradbury H, Reason P (eds) 2000 Handbook of action research. Sage, Thousand Oaks, CA
Braud W, Anderson R (eds) 1998 Transpersonal research methods for the social sciences: honoring human experience. Sage, Thousand Oaks, CA
Brockman J (ed) 1977 About Bateson. Dutton, New York
Carr W, Kemmis S 1986 Becoming critical: education, knowledge and action research. Falmer, Basingstoke, Hants
Clements J, Ettling D, Jenett D, Shields L 1998 Organic research: feminine spirituality meets transpersonal research. In: Braud W, Anderson R (eds) Transpersonal research methods for the social sciences: honoring human experience. Sage, Thousand Oaks, CA
Cooperrider D L, Srivastva S 1987 Appreciative inquiry in organizational life. In: Woodman R, Pasmore W (eds) Research in organizational change and development, vol 1. JAI, Greenwich
Cousins N 1990 Head first: the biology of hope and the healing power of the human spirit. Penguin, New York
de Cuevas J 1995 The pleasing placebo (article on the internet, copyright President and Fellows of Harvard College)
Fals-Borda O, Rahman M A (eds) 1991 Action and knowledge: breaking the monopoly with participatory action research. Intermediate Technology/Apex, New York
Fryer D, Feather N T 1994 Intervention techniques, qualitative methods in organizational research. Sage, London
Gergen K J 1973 Social psychology as history. Journal of Personality and Social Psychology 26:309–320
Goleman D 1996 Emotional intelligence. Bloomsbury, London
Guba E G, Lincoln Y S 1989 Fourth generation evaluation. Sage, Newbury Park, CA
Guba E G, Lincoln Y S 1994 Competing paradigms in qualitative research. In: Denzin N K, Lincoln Y S (eds) Handbook of qualitative research. Sage, Thousand Oaks, CA
Harré R, Secord P F 1972 The explanation of social behaviour. Basil Blackwell, Oxford
Heather N 1976 Radical perspectives in psychology. Methuen, London
Heron J 1971 Experience and method. University of Surrey, Guildford
Heron J 1981a Philosophical basis for a new paradigm. In: Reason P, Rowan J (eds) Human inquiry: a sourcebook of new paradigm research. John Wiley, Chichester

Heron J 1981b Experiential research methodology. In: Reason P, Rowan J (eds) Human inquiry: a sourcebook of new paradigm research. John Wiley, Chichester

Heron J 1985 The role of reflection in cooperative inquiry. In: Boud D, Keogh R, Walker D (eds) Reflection: turning experience into learning. Kogan Page, London

Heron J 1986 Critique of conventional research methodology. Complementary Medical Research 1(1):12–22

Heron J 1988 Validity in co-operative inquiry. In: Reason P (ed) Human inquiry in action. Sage, London

Heron J 1992 Feeling and personhood: psychology in another key. Sage, London

Heron J 1996 Co-operative inquiry: research into the human condition. Sage, London

Heron J 1998 Sacred science: person-centred inquiry into the spiritual and the subtle. PCCS, Ross-on-Wye, Herefordshire

Heron J 2000 Transpersonal co-operative inquiry. In: Bradbury H, Reason P (eds) Handbook of action research. Sage, Thousand Oaks, CA;

Heron J, Reason P 1985 Whole person medicine: a co-operative inquiry. British Postgraduate Medical Federation, London

Heron J, Reason P 1986 Research with people. Person-centered Review 4(1):456–476

Heron J, Reason P 1997 A participatory inquiry paradigm. Qualitative Inquiry 3(3):274–294

Heron J, Reason P 2000 Co-operative inquiry. In: Bradbury H, Reason P (eds) Handbook of action research. Sage, Thousand Oaks, CA;

Israel J, Tajfel H (eds) 1972 The context of social psychology: a critical assessment. Academic Press, New York

Joynson R B 1974 Psychology and common sense. Routledge & Kegan Paul, London

Kelly G B 1993 Karl Rahner: theologian of the graced search for meaning. Clark, Edinburgh

Lincoln Y S, Guba E G 1985 Naturalistic inquiry. Sage, Beverly Hills, CA

Merleau-Ponty M 1962 Phenomenology of perception. Routledge & Kegan Paul, London

Mies X 1993

Olesen V 1994 Feminisms and models of qualitative research. In: Denzin N K, Lincoln Y S (eds) Handbook of qualitative research. Sage, Thousand Oaks, CA

Reason P 1986 Innovative research techniques. Complementary Medical Research 1(1):23–39

Reason P 1988a (ed) Human inquiry in action. Sage, London

Reason P 1988b Whole person medical practice. In: Reason P (ed) Human inquiry in action. Sage, London

Reason P 1991 Power and conflict in multi-disciplinary collaboration. Complementary Medical Research 5(3):144–150

Reason P 1994a (ed) Participation in human inquiry. Sage, London

Reason P 1994b Three approaches to participative inquiry. In: Denzin N K, Lincoln Y S (eds) Handbook of qualitative research. Sage, Thousand Oaks, CA

Reason P, Heron J 1986 The human capacity for intentional self-healing and enhanced wellness: a research proposal. British Journal of Holistic Medicine 1(2):123–134

Reason P, Heron J 1995 Co-operative inquiry. In: Smith J A, Harré R, Van Langenhove L (eds) Rethinking methods in psychology. Sage, London

Reason P, Rowan J 1981 (eds) Human inquiry: a sourcebook of new paradigm research. John Wiley, Chichester

Schön D 1983 The reflective practitioner: how professionals think in action. Basic Books, New York

Shotter J 1975 Images of man in psychological research. Methuen, London

Skolimowski H 1994 The participatory mind. Arkana, London

Smith J A, Harré R, Van Langenhove L (eds) 1995 Rethinking psychology. Sage, London

Spiegel D 1993 Living beyond limits: new hope and help for facing life threatening illness. Vermillion, London

Spretnak C 1991 States of grace: the recovery of meaning in the postmodern age. HarperCollins, New York

Torbert W R 1991 The power of balance: transforming self, society and scientific inquiry. Sage, Newbury Park, CA

Varela F, Thompson E, Rosch E 1993 The embodied mind. MIT, Cambridge, MA

Watkins A (ed) 1997 Mind–body medicine: a clinician's guide to psychoneuroimmunology. Churchill Livingstone, New York

Weinstein J 1974 Allocation of subjects in medical experiments. New England Journal of Medicine 291:1278–1285

Epilogue

13

Psychoneuroimmunology: the mind–brain connection

Peter Fenwick

Editor's note

Professor Fenwick is a neuropsychiatrist. Nevertheless (or perhaps because of this), I gave him the last word on the death of the mind–body split. I asked him to to go beyond the evidence for mind–body interaction and to speculate about a more mysterious entanglement of one consciousness with another. Peter touches on studies of prayer and instant healing, a now fashionable research area where the evidence though so far inconclusive in nevertheless tantalising. Do para-psychological or prayer studies support the idea that we affect one another not only when face to face, not just through touch and relationship but through non-located consciousness? This would pitch us into the vertiginous perspectives of a profoundly participatory cosmos, where consciousness no longer obeys the laws of time and space. This sounds like familiar territory; not one associated with science, but rather with the trans-personal, the spiritual and the super-natural. Yet the emerging science of consciousness may yet reveal a common basis for phenomena like intuition, synchronicity, unexplained remission and healing at a distance. If emerging ideas about non-located consciousness eventually provide a radical (and radically dis-embodied) theory about how we affect one another, it will be the ultimate step in rehabilitating the so-called placebo response.

It takes only a moment's self-observation to recognize that what goes on in the mind must affect the body. If you look out at a gentle seascape you will begin to feel relaxed and tranquil, whereas coping with the hassle on the tube in London is likely to generate stress and anxiety. The mind and body are closely coupled together. Many Eastern therapeutic traditions go beyond this as they argue that humans are embedded in the matrix of the universe and that the universe influences body and mind together.

Regarding either body or mind as an entity on its own gives only part of the picture. Qigong, a Chinese philosophical system, argues that the rhythmic pulse of nature throughout the 24 hours makes itself manifest in the rhythms of the body. There are thus particular times during the day when certain actions should be undertaken, and this is reflected in a more limited way in Western medicine today, in for example the sleep/alertness cycle. Ancient wisdom goes beyond that because it recognizes that the natural flowing of energies through the body can be life enhancing and that if their flow is restricted it can lead to illness.

Our Western culture has a long history, dating back to the time of the Greeks, of a recognition of the relationship between mind and body. Galen (130 AD) the Greek philosopher noticed that melancholy women were more susceptible to breast cancer than were sanguine women. Thus much of our allopathic medicine in the West is covertly based on an acceptance that mind and brain interact. It was not until the 1930s when psychology wished to ignore mind that the major difficulties for mind–body medicine arose. In the 1950s and 60s early studies were beginning to produce evidence that those who were under stress were more likely to become ill. It seems that the Romans and the public schools were indeed correct in observing *mens sana in corpore sano*.

Solomon & Moos in 1964 suggested that this relationship between mind or psychological processes and the response of the body to stress should be termed psychoimmunology. As the scientific work in this area was extended it became clear that this view was too limited, because many of the responses were mediated by brain function. Ader (1990) proposed the word psychoneuroimmunology (PNI) and this has generally been accepted. There have been several definitions of PNI but the one that is normally used is *the study of the intricate interaction of consciousness (psycho) brain and central nervous system (neuro) and the body's defence against infection and abnormal cell division (immunology)*. There has been a rapid growth in this field and books on mind–body medicine are now being published at regular intervals.

In my own field of epilepsy the relationship between mind and brain is very clear. It is now well recognized that seizures may be caused by stressful events in a patient's life. Seizures do not just occur because the anticonvulsants are too low or there is some progression in the underlying epileptic pathology although, of course, this may be so. Frequently they occur because of an interaction between patients and the circumstances in their life. In one study that we carried out at the Maudsley Hospital over 50% of patients reported having seizures when they were angry, upset, tired and under stress. Most of the patients saw happiness as a very powerful anticonvulsant. Only 4% had seizures when they were happy.

This chapter will look at some brain–body mechanisms that are important in health and disease. This area of research is now rapidly advancing so it is not possible to give more than a flavour of some of the important areas. However, there are a number of books for interested readers who would like to take their knowledge further.

UPWARD AND DOWNWARD CAUSATION

Our current medicine is based on reductionism—the scientific world view that simple processes give rise to more complex ones. In medicine it is the physics of the atoms and molecules that leads to the formation of chemical compounds. The theory of chemistry describes how chemicals combine in various ways to make the proteins, which are the basis of biology. Biology describes how these basic proteins form the cells and how cell structure is dependent entirely on these proteins. The DNA of the chromosome directs the functioning of cellular structures and determines how they will organize together in groups. Fluctuations in health are seen in our current medical model as flowing from these simple basic processes. Infection is regarded as being due to an infecting organism outwitting the mechanism of immunity. Cardiovascular disease is seen as the occurrence of fatty plaques, atheroma, in the vessel walls. This view of science and medicine suggests that upward causation from the simplest structures to the more complex is the way that the world is organized, but this is a view that is increasingly being challenged. Science has been concerned with upward causation for so long that it finds difficulty in seeing that macroscopic events within a biological system (in this case mind and meaning) may play a major part in the organization of and may direct the physics, chemistry and biology of lower-order systems.

This control by higher-order systems of lower-order systems within the body is called 'downward causation'. Control is thought to go from mind (including social and cultural meaning) through the central nervous system to bodily function. Roger Sperry in 1987 pointed out that downward causation within the central nervous system is a common property 'things are controlled not only from below upwards but also from above downwards by mental … and other macro properties (furthermore) primacy is given to the highest level control rather than the lowest (Sperry 1987)'. Downward causation is coming to be recognized as an important branch of mind–body medicine. It is now agreed that what we think and feel alters the body's functioning.

There is, however, still considerable resistance to this concept. Willis Harman, writing in the *New Metaphysical Foundations of Modern Science* (1994), says:

Scientists too quickly assume (or behave as though they do) that the philosophical premises underlying science are not at issue—but they are part of the definition of modern science … Yet many debates that appear to be about scientific matters in fact centre around implicit ontological issues about the ultimate nature of reality, and the epistemological issues about how we might find out.

Thus often the issue is not about macro-organization within the central nervous system influencing lower-order processes, but about the extent to which mind itself is able to alter the body's biology. Lawrence Foss (1994) has written on this subject. Postmodernist science is already being forced to acknowledge that complex systems may not be entirely controlled by the smallest elements. There is now evidence that complex systems can be self-organizing and that very small changes in the dynamics of the system can lead to the emergence of quite new organizing principles.

It is thus important to recognize that downward causation may be a fundamental property of the central nervous system and that thoughts, feelings, meanings, desires, etc. are organizing principles that lead to the emergence of control functions within the body as a whole. The new science of PNI is one such attempt to investigate and formulate these principles.

So far we have discussed only mind and its possible relevance to modification of bodily pathology. However, there is beyond this a possibility that mind itself, or certainly consciousness, is a widely distributed property and that in some way it contributes to the organizing principle, which may lie outside and beyond the brain. A number of philosophical systems support this view.

THE IMMUNE SYSTEM

An excellent overview of the immune system is given by J. McDaniel (1996). The function of the immune system is to protect the body both from outside infections and from its own cells that are functioning abnormally (tumours). In order to do this it has to be able to differentiate those proteins that arise from within the body from those arising from outside. This function is carried out essentially by the lymphocytes, some of which are concerned with humoral immunity (circulating antibodies), the B lymphocytes, and others with cell-mediated immunity, the T lymphocytes.

In cell-mediated immunity T lymphocytes are directly involved in the immune response. Cellular immunity is mainly mediated by three subgroups of T lymphocytes, helper T cells, cytotoxic T cells and suppressor T cells. Each has a specific function: helper T cells augment cellular and humoral responses by lymphokines, cytotoxic T cells directly attack and destroy target antigen cells and suppressor T cells, through negative feedback, autoregulate the immune response.

Humoral immunity is produced by circulating antibodies, which are produced by the B lymphocytes. These antibodies (immunoglobulins) fall into five major categories IgG, IgM, IgA, IgE and IgD and they protect the body from being invaded by bacterial toxins and encapsulated bacteria.

A new population of cells known as non-B and non-T lymphocytes has recently been discovered. These are known as natural killer (NK) cells and they are thought to be involved in the defence against neoplastic growth and metastases and some viral infection. These cells can be activated without an antigen and they are thought to be involved in many of the processes due to PNI.

EFFECTS OF EVERYDAY STRESSFUL EVENTS

It is impossible to lead an ordinary life without being stressed, sometimes severely. Medical students report more illnesses associated with exam periods than at other times (Glaser et al 1987). Second-year medical students undergoing exam stress have also shown declines in NK-cell activity, with a reduction in alternations in cellular antiviral and antitumour activity (Kiecolt-Glaser et al 1984). Another study by Dorian et al (1982) showed that in a group of psychiatry residents, compared with age and sex-matched physician controls, there were higher levels of emotional distress before the examinations and a reduction in mytogen-induced lymphocyte proliferation and slightly higher numbers of T and B lymphocytes.

It has been recognized for some time that high life-event scores are related to an increased frequency not only of depressive illness, but also of physical illness. Locke et al (1989) found low rates of NK-cell activity were associated with high life-event scores and stress symptoms. It is of interest that NK-cell activity was normal if there were high life-event scores but no subjective feelings of stress. Sleep deprivation and stress in psychological tests were also found to produce immune response changes (Landman et al 1984).

In an interesting review Hillhouse & Adler (1996) point to the significance of continuous persistent stress. They report the work of Kiecolt-Glaser et al (1988, 1991) who showed that caregivers looking after demented relatives, compared with matched controls, showed significantly greater emotional distress and poor immune functioning. The total number of T lymphocytes and T-helper cells were reduced, with an increase in Epstein–Barr virus titres. Those who were under long-term stress showed down-regulation on three measures of cellular immunity and the caregivers also reported significantly more days' infectious illness. An interesting study is that of individuals living near the Three Mile Island nuclear power plant (Gatchell et al 1985). They found that, compared with controls, the residents had fewer T lymphocytes, T-helper and T-suppressor cells. This has been confirmed by other studies that have shown fewer NK cells.

THE PROTECTIVE VALUE OF OPTIMISM

It does matter how we see our lives, and whether we look forward to the future optimistically, or whether we feel so trodden down that the future is unattractive. A notable long-term study was carried out by Peterson and his colleagues over a period of 35 years. The Harvard study of Adult Development chose 268 men from Harvard in 1942 to 1944. They were chosen because of their good physical and psychological health and high level of academic success. These men had been in the war and were asked to write about their war experiences and how successful they had been with their commanders, men under them, and what their own opinion of themselves was. These essays were then rated so as to extract their score on a scale that ranged from extreme optimism to extreme pessimism. Correlations with their health over the years showed that those who scored optimistically at the beginning of the study were healthier later in life than men who had more pessimistic ratings (Peterson & Bossio 1993). This correlation became strongest at the age of 45, two decades after the optimism was assessed. So clearly, how you approach life makes a difference.

A second study by these authors looked at a group of 172 undergraduates in 1994. Questionnaires estimated their level of optimism and the number of days of illness that they had had during the previous month. One year later it was found that the more optimistic students had fewer days of illness and had fewer doctor visits than did the more pessimistic students. The authors note that the reduction of illness in the optimistic group suggests an influence of optimism on the immune system. This possibility of a strengthened immune system was investigated by Kamen-Siegel et al (1991) in a study of 47 subjects rated for their level of optimism. The more optimistic individuals had higher helper/suppressor cell ratios (helper T cells and suppressor T cells) suggesting that their immune system was better able to combat disease.

There is also evidence from other studies. In one study women with breast cancer who were optimistic lived longer than others in the sample (Levy et al 1991). Another study followed 160 men who had suffered one heart attack for 8 years. At the end of the study, 60 had died; those surviving had been rated as optimistic at the beginning of the study (Buchanan & Seligman 1995).

In a study by Pennebaker, Kiecolt-Glaser & Glaser (1988) 50 healthy undergraduates were asked to write about either traumatic events that they had experienced or ordinary everyday topics for four consecutive days. The hypothesis was that traumatic events that were not disclosed were likely to prove stressful, whereas writing about them was likely to reduce stress. The immediate results were that trauma writers noted some negative short-term emotional reactions, but after 6 months they appeared to be happier and less depressed than the controls. There was some evidence that disclosing trauma enhanced immune system activity and there was also evidence that those who wrote about trauma had a drop in visits to the health centre during the study period of 6 weeks as opposed to the controls.

The authors note that there was no conclusive evidence that improved immune function correlated with improved health, but the data pointed this way.

PSYCHOSOCIAL INTERVENTIONS

A study by Fawzy et al (1993) looked at the intervention of group therapy in patients who had had a malignant melanoma removed. The follow-up in this study had continued for more than 6 years. After surgical treatment the subjects were randomized to a control group and to a structured psychiatric intervention consisting of six weekly one-and-a-half-hour group sessions. In these sessions, stress management was taught as were general coping skills and behaviours. There were also psychological sessions, which were designed to alter the emotional reaction to cancer. The experimenters measured emotional reactions and coping skills, the patients' health, cancer recurrence and survival times. There were also frequent immunological assays. They found that a high baseline of distress predicted better survival and recurrence rates (were those with initial low distress in denial?). At 6 years' postintervention the treatment group had significantly better survival and a trend for longer time to recurrence than controls. Changes in coping skills predicted a better survival time, although, surprisingly, changes in total mood did not. The percentage of NK cells and interferon-augmented NK-cell activity was associated with lower depression and anxiety and an increase in anger.

In an ongoing study the relationship between mood—depression and anger—was studied by Keller et al (1992) in a group of 300 inner city adolescents. The intake to this study comprised healthy adolescents recruited from local high schools, or depressed adolescents with depressed mood or clinical depression, recruited from an adolescent medicine clinic. They found an interesting relationship in that those depressed at intake had had more physical illnesses 9 months later. There was an association between high depression levels at intake and some immune system markers. Of further interest was the finding that high levels of anger at intake showed a relationship with an increase in upper respiratory tract infections, and a decreased white blood cell count. However, further analysis of this group showed that if the anger was directed towards others as verbal aggression there was an improvement in immunity with fewer illnesses. Conversely, aggression directed against the self (psychoanalytical depression) was associated with a reduced immune response (decreased T cells) and an increase in all infections.

It is clear that marriages can either be highly successful and supportive, when the married couple is happy and relaxed, or they can be the source of enormous emotional stress. Kielcolt-Glaser et al (1987, 1988) in two small studies found that lower marital satisfaction was associated with poorer immune functioning as well as greater depression and loneliness. A more comprehensive study used 19 newly-wed couples and demographically appropriate couples without children who had obtained their marriage licence 4 to 6 months prior to the study. All couples were given a 30-minute interview to discuss areas of disagreement, and this session was rated for problem-solving behaviour, emotion expressed, etc. A blood sample after this episode showed that hostile behaviour during marital conflict was associated with decreased levels of prolactin, and increased levels of growth hormone, adrenocorticotrophic hormone (ACTH), adrenaline and noradrenaline. The high levels of adrenaline and noradrenaline lead to down-regulation of the immunological system and thus it is likely that this group was more immunologically compromised. Prolactin, on the other hand, was enhanced in the low-hostility group, and prolactin is known to be immune enhancing. Other immune function markers also suggested that the high-hostility group had suppression of immune function. Women whose husbands were more likely to withdraw follow-ing their wives' negative behaviours were more likely to show immune system compromise, whereas the husbands' immune systems were not compromised.

These gender differences have also been found in other studies. An interesting study relates to hypertension in middle-aged married couples (average age 57). The wives showed larger blood pressure increases during marital conflict than the husbands. The women's blood pressure changes were related to marital quality and hostile behaviour. The men's blood pressure increases were related only to speech rate.

It is now common knowledge that there is a relationship between stress and viral infection. However, it is difficult to assess exactly how secure the data are. A study in the Medical Research Council's Common Cold Unit between 1986 and 1989 (Cohen, Tyrrell & Smith 1993) is one of the best prospective studies. Here subjects were assessed for stressful life events, perceived stresses and negative affect before they were experimentally exposed to the common cold virus; 154 men and 266 women volunteered. The results showed that more highly stressed people have higher rates of cold irrespective of the stress scale used, and this was not because people who were highly stressed were indulging in addictive antihealth behaviour such as drinking, smoking, etc. There was also no correlation with person-ality factors. It was found that the relationship between life events and colds was independent of the relation between both perceived stress and clinical illness, and negative affect and clinical illness, so each contributed. The important finding from this study was that just experiencing signifi-cant life events was sufficient to increase your rate of illness independent of whether the life event itself was felt as stressful, and whether or not it evoked a negative affect.

GUIDED IMAGERY

A number of studies have looked at the efficacy of treating patients suffering from cancer with guided imagery. The subject is a complex one, as simply coming into a study can itself change levels of optimism and social responsiveness, and these are both confounding factors. Although it has been shown that guided imagery patients may improve, there has been little evidence to support the contention that this effect has been mediated by the changes in immune system functioning. Gruber et al 1988 assessed the impact of guided imagery on 10 patients with cancer. They were five male and five female patients ranging in age from 34 to 69 years, and they had different forms of metastatic disease. All subjects were medically and psychiatrically stable and none were familiar with the use of imagery in relaxation. Each subject acted as their own control.

The results of this study showed that there were significant changes in immune system responsiveness. Total plasma levels of IgM and IgG increased significantly during the study period. There were also significant increases in NK-cell activity and responsiveness of peripheral blood lymphocytes to T-cell mitogens, but no changes were seen in total IgA levels. It could be argued that these changes were not related to the clinical improvement noted in patients carrying out guided imagery. However, there are clear changes in immune system function with guided imagery, and it is reasonable to assume that they are correlated.

DOWNWARD CAUSATION, PRAYER AND INTERCONNECTEDNESS

This chapter so far has demonstrated a significant effect of downward causation in the nervous system. Meaning is important, and the negative interpretation given to events leads to a reduction in immune system responsiveness and effectiveness. Thus, avoiding life events, positive affective response to circumstances, loving supportive relationships, optimism for the future and learning how to cope with psychological stresses can all modify immune system activity, and so reduce the rate of infection or the rate of cancer progression. Clearly, a healthy well-balanced mind is supportive of a healthy well-balanced immune system.

So far we have considered only our current scientific view that psychological processes are generated entirely within the brain and limited to the brain and the organism. Over the last 50 years large numbers of parapsychological experiments have been carried out suggesting that the mind is not limited to the skull and that it is possible to demonstrate the effect of mind on other minds (telepathy) and the effect of mind on matter (psychokinesis). For those interested in a more comprehensive review of this subject, the recent book by Dean Radin, *The Conscious Universe*, provides a wide range of references to the studies and examines some of the meta-analyses that have demonstrated these effects.

Our current physics through the study of quantum mechanical effects suggests that the universe is highly interconnected and that particles interact with each other at a distance. Thus the idea that mind could also be interactive outside the skull is theoretically possible although at the present time the mechanism by which this could occur is not yet known.

Some support for this view is given by a number of studies that have shown a significant effect of healing at a distance both by the use of non-contact healing, and by prayer. However, the recent Cochrane report on the healing effects of prayer could not demonstrate a convincing significant effect, but found only three controlled trials in the literature. Their conclusion was that, although there is no evidence for prayer, there is also no evidence against prayer and thus it is reasonable to continue using prayer until such a time as further studies have been conducted that clarify the position.

Gardner (1983) in a delightful paper in the Christmas issue of the British Medical Journal, looks at the effects of prayer on healing as is reported to have been carried out by St Cuthbert. He also adds several anecdotal cases of his own in which prayer has been responsible for miraculous cures.

In contrast to the paucity of good evidence for prayer on people, there are a number of studies that have been well carried out and show a significant effect of non-contact healing, or healing at a distance (prayer), on a wide range of biological systems: yeasts, enzymes, fungi, red blood cells, grass and vegetables. Benor reviewed 131 controlled trials of which 56 were significant at $P < 0.01$, and 21 significant at $P > 0.02$ and $P < 0.05$ (Benor 1993).

Benor also reviewed non-contact healing, or healing at a distance (prayer), in humans. He found 32 controlled trials that have been properly conducted. Of these 15 showed a significant beneficial effect of healing at a significance of $P < 0.01$. These studies showed improvements in pain, hypertension, asthma, coronary heart disease, skin wound healing, haemoglobin increase, headaches and anxiety.

There is thus evidence that mind can produce effects outside the skull, leading to the conclusion that downward causation not only occurs from individual mind to individual brain but also from other minds to other brains. The strength of this more general effect would seem to be weak but is nevertheless present. A healing encounter will thus take place at many different levels.

CONCLUSION

This chapter review the evidence for the effects of downward causation on the genesis of illness and healing in humans. There is a large body of knowledge giving a detailed picture of the human immune system and its method of functioning. This picture now includes the way that the immune system is modified by psychological processes, and it details how meaning, loving or stressful relationships can alter our state of health. Components of the biological pathway for the effects of hope or pessimism have been defined.

Of more importance, there is also evidence that humans may no longer remain an island, but are interconnected with their fellow humans in a clearly demonstrable way. Non-contact healing and healing at a distance occurs. Prayer has been shown to be effective. This leads to the conclusion that what we think matters at two levels: first, because of downward causation within our own central nervous system, and, secondly, through its weak but present direct effect on the brains of other people.

REFERENCES

Ader R, Felten D, Cohen N (eds) 1990 Psychoneuroimmunology (2nd ed) Academic Press, San Diego

Bachan E, Manuck S, Cohen S et al 1994 Adrenergic blockade ameliorates cellular immune responses to mental stress in humans (submitted for publication)

Benor D 1993 Healing research. Helix, Munich

Buchanan GM, Seligman MEP (eds) 1995 Explanatory style. Lawrence Erlbaum Associates, Hillsdale, NJ, pp ix, 303

Cohen S, Tyrrell D, Smith AP 1993 Negative life events, perceived stress, negative affect, and susceptibility to the common cold. Journal of Personality and Social Psychology 64: 131–140

Coleman D, Gurin J (eds) 1993 Mind body medicine. Consumer Reports Books, New York

Dorian B, Garfinkle P, Keystone E, Gorczynski R, Darby P 1986 Stress immunity and illness. Psychosomatic Medicine 48: 304–305

Fawzy I, Fawzy N, Hyun C et al 1993 Malignant melanoma: effects of early structured psychiatric intervention, coping, and effective state on recurrence and survival six years later. Arch. Gen. Psych. 50: 681–689

Foss et al 1994 The biomedical paradigm, psychoneuroimmunology, and the black four of hearts. Advances 10: 1

Gardner R 1983 Modern miracles. British Medical Journal (Christmas issue) 1983

Gatchel RJ, Schaeffer MA, Baum A 1985 A psychological field study of stress at Three Mile Island. Psychophysiology 22(2): 175–181

Glaser R, Rice J, Sheridan J et al 1987 Stress related immune suppression: health implications. Brain Behaviour and Immunity 1: 7–20

Gruber B, Hall N, Hersh S, Dubois P 1988 Immune system and psychological changes in metastatic cancer patients while using ritulised relaxation and guided imagery: a pilot study. Scandanavian Journal of Behaviour Therapy 17: 25–46

Harman W 1994 A re-examination of the metaphysical foundations of modern science. Why is it necessary? In: Harman W (ed) New metaphysical foundations of modern science. Institute of Noetic Sciences

Hillhouse JJ, Adler CM 1996 Evaluating a simple model of work stress, burnout, affective and physical symptoms in hospital nurses. Psychology, Health & Medicine 1(3): 297–306

Kamen-Siegel L, Rodin J, Seligman M, Dwyer J 1991 Explanatory style and cell mediated immunity in elderly men and women. Health Psychology 10: 229–235

Keller S, Schleifer S, Bartlett J, Eckholdt H 1992 Affective processes and immune dysfunction have health consequences. Biological Psychiatry 31: 236A

Kiecolt-Glaser J, Garner W, Speicher C, Penn G, Holiday J, Glaser R 1984. Psychosocial modifiers of immuno competence in medical students. Psychosomatic Medicine 46: 7–14

Kiecolt-Glaser J, Glaser R 1988 Methodological issues in behavioural immunology research with humans. Brain Behaviour and Immunity 2: 67–78

Kiecolt-Glaser J, Fisher L, Ogrocki P, Sout J, Speicher C, Glaser R 1987 Marital quality, marital disruption, and immune function. Psychosomatic Medicine 49: 13–33

Kiecolt-Glaser J, Kennedy S, Malkoff S, Fisher L, Speicher C, Glaser R 1988 Marital discord and immunity in males. Psychosomatic Medicine 50: 213–229

Kiecolt-Glaser J, Dura J, Speicher C, Trask O, Glaser R 1991 Spousal caregivers of dementia victims. Longitudinal changes in immunity and health. Psychosomatic Medicine 53: 345–362

Levy S, Herberman R, Lippmann M, d'Angelo T, Lee J 1991 Immunological and psychosocial predictors of disease. Recurrence in patients with early stage breast cancer. Behavioural Medicine 17: 67–75

Locke S, Kraus L, Lesserman J, Hurst M, Heisel S, Williams R 1984 Life change stress, psychiatric symptoms, and natural killer cell activity. Psychosomatic Medicine 46: 441–453

Landman R, Muller F, Perrini C, Wesp M, Erne P, Buhler F 1984 Changes of immuno-regulatory cells induced by psychophysiological and physical stress: relationship to plasma catecholamines. Clinical and Experimental Immunology 58: 127–135

Locke SE, Colligan D 1986 The healer within: the new medicine of mind and body. E. P. Dutton, New York, NY p. xvi

McDaniel JS 1996 Stressful life events and psychoneuroimmunology. In: Miller TW et al (ed) Theory and assessment of stressful life events. International Universities Press Stress and Health Series. International Universities Press, Madison, CT pp 3–36

Pennebaker J, Kiecolt-Glaser J, Glaser R 1988 Disclosure of traumas and immune function: health implications for psychotherapy. Journal of Consulting and Clinical Psychology 50: 213–229

Peterson C, Bossio L 1993 Healthy attitudes: optimism, hope, and control. In: Goldman D, Gurin J (eds) Mind body medicine. Consumer Reports Books, pp 351–366

Rabin B, Kusnecov A, Shurin M, Zhou D, Rasnick S 1994 Mechanistic aspects of stressor induced immune alteration. In: Glazier R, Keicolt-Glazier J (eds) Handbook of human stress and immunity. Academic Press, London, pp 23–51

Radin D 1997 The conscious universe. Harper *Edge*, San Francisco

Schedlowski M, Jacobs R, Stratmann G et al 1993 Changes of natural killer cells during acute psychological stress. Journal of Clinical Immunology 13: 119–126

Solomon GF, Moos R 1964 Emotions, immunity, and disease. Archives of General Psychiatry 11(6): 657–674

Sperry RW 1987 Structure and significance of the consciousness revolution. The Journal of Mind and Behaviour 8: 1

Index